Treatment-resistant Depression

Treatment-resistant Depression

Edited by

Siegfried Kasper, MD

Professor and Chair, Department of Psychiatry and Psychotherapy, Medical University of Vienna, Vienna, Austria

Stuart Montgomery, MD

Emeritus Professor of Psychiatry, Professor of Psychiatry (retired), Imperial College of Science, Technology and Medicine, University of London, London, UK

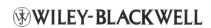

A John Wiley & Sons, Ltd., Publication

This edition first published 2013, © 2013 by John Wiley & Sons, Ltd

Wiley-Blackwell is an imprint of John Wiley & Sons, formed by the merger of Wiley's global Scientific, Technical and Medical business with Blackwell Publishing.

Registered Office
John Wiley & Sons, Ltd, The Atrium, Southern Gate, Chichester, West Sussex, PO19 8SQ, UK

Editorial Offices
9600 Garsington Road, Oxford, OX4 2DQ, UK
The Atrium, Southern Gate, Chichester, West Sussex, PO19 8SQ, UK
2121 State Avenue, Ames, Iowa 50014-8300, USA

For details of our global editorial offices, for customer services and for information about how to apply for permission to reuse the copyright material in this book please see our website at www.wiley.com/wiley-blackwell.

The right of the author to be identified as the author of this work has been asserted in accordance with the UK Copyright, Designs and Patents Act 1988.

Library of Congress Cataloging-in-Publication Data

Treatment-resistant depression / [edited by] Siegfried Kasper, Stuart Montgomery.
      p. ; cm.
   Includes bibliographical references and index.
   ISBN 978-1-119-95290-9 (pbk.)
I. Kasper, S. (Siegfried)   II. Montgomery, S. A.
[DNLM: 1. Depressive Disorder, Treatment-Resistant–therapy.
2. Antidepressive Agents–therapeutic use.   3. Psychotherapy. WM 171.5]
   616.85′2706–dc23

                                                    2012043215

A catalogue record for this book is available from the British Library.

Wiley also publishes its books in a variety of electronic formats. Some content that appears in print may not be available in electronic books.

Cover image: © Mike Kiev, iStockphoto.com.
Cover design by Sarah Dickinson.

Set in 10.5/12.5pt Times by SPi Publisher Services, Pondicherry, India
Printed and bound in Malaysia by Vivar Printing Sdn Bhd

1   2013

Contents

List of Contributors

Dr. Elena Akimova, MD   Department of Psychiatry and Psychotherapy, Medical University of Vienna, Vienna, Austria

Prof. Michael Bauer, MD, PhD   Professor and Chair of Psychiatry, Department of Psychiatry and Psychotherapy, University Hospital Carl Gustav Carus, Dresden University of Technology, Dresden, Germany

Dr. Chiara Fabbri, MD   Department of Biomedical and NeuroMotor Sciences, University of Bologna, Bologna, Italy

Dr. Ramesh K. Gupta, MD   Consultation and Liaison Psychiatry Unit, The Canberra Hospital, Canberra, Australia

Dr. Robert Haußmann, MD   Department of Psychiatry and Psychotherapy, University Hospital Carl Gustav Carus, Dresden University of Technology, Dresden, Germany

Prof. Siegfried Kasper, MD   Professor and Chair, Department of Psychiatry and Psychotherapy, Medical University of Vienna, Vienna, Austria

Dr. Sarah Kayser, MD, MSc   Department of Psychiatry and Psychotherapy, University Hospital Bonn, Bonn, Germany

Prof. Hans-Jürgen Möller, MD   Professor Emeritus and former Chair of Psychiatry, Department of Psychiatry and Psychotherapy, Ludwig Maximilians University, Munich, Germany

Prof. Stuart Montgomery, MD   Emeritus Professor of Psychiatry, Professor of Psychiatry (retired), Imperial College of Science, Technology and Medicine, University of London, London, UK

Prof. William Pitchot, MD, PhD   Department of Psychiatry, University of Liège, Liège, Belgium

Dr. Stefano Porcelli, MD   Department of Biomedical and NeuroMotor Sciences, University of Bologna, Bologna, Italy

Dr. Rebecca Schennach, MD   Department of Psychiatry and Psychotherapy, Ludwig Maximilians University, Munich, Germany

Prof. Thomas E. Schläpfer, MD   Vice Chair and Professor of Psychiatry and Psychotherapy, Department of Psychiatry and Psychotherapy, University Hospital Bonn, Bonn, Germany; Associate Professor of Psychiatry and Mental Health, The Johns Hopkins University School of Medicine, Maryland, USA

Dr. Florian Seemüller, MD   Department of Psychiatry and Psychotherapy, Ludwig Maximilians University, Munich, Germany

Prof. Alessandro Serretti, MD, PhD   Department of Biomedical and NeuroMotor Sciences, University of Bologna, Bologna, Italy

Prof. Daniel Souery, MD   Director at Psy Pluriel, European Centre of Psychological Medicine – PsyPluriel, Brussels, Belgium

Prof. Michael E. Thase, MD   Professor Psychiatry, Perelman School of Medicine, University of Pennsylvania, Philadelphia Veterans Affairs Medical Center, PA, USA; Adjunct Professor of Psychiatry, University of Pittsburgh Medical Center, PA, USA

Foreword

Clinical depression is both a symptom and a debilitating disorder. The World Bank estimates that, by 2020, depression will become the most common noncommunicable disease in the world, with the heaviest burden of disease. Depression carries with it stigma, and the disease is misunderstood as a lack of will power. The proven strategies for treating depression include both pharmacotherapy and psychotherapy, as well as a mixture of the two.

Treatment-resistant depression remains relatively common and the reasons for this vary from missing diagnoses to inadequate therapeutic interventions. Definitions of treatment-resistant depression also vary. Treatment-resistant depression can be a staging process, which can enable clinicians to intervene appropriately and adequately, so that the burden of the disease is reduced and quality of life for the patient and their carers can be improved. Investigations for staging models must include both biological and nonbiological factors. In addition, cultural variations must be taken into account. Psychotherapy alone or in combination with pharmacotherapy is part of the therapeutic armamentarium.

The editors, both eminent psychiatrists in the field, with international reputations, have brought together a star-studded cast to explain not only the staging process but interventions too, making this volume of great interest and much use for clinicians in their clinical practice. For this alone, the editors deserve our congratulations and thanks.

Dinesh Bhugra CBE
Professor of Mental Health & Cultural Diversity
Institute of Psychiatry, King's College London
President-Elect, World Psychiatric Association

CHAPTER 1

Definitions and Predictors of Treatment-resistant Depression

Daniel Souery

European Centre of Psychological Medicine – PsyPluriel, Brussels, Belgium

William Pitchot

Department of Psychiatry, University of Liège, Liège, Belgium

Summary

Treatment-resistant depression (TRD) remains a common condition, with 50–60% of patients not achieving meaningful response following antidepressant treatment. The huge complexity of the phenomenon and the wide variety of parameters that must be taken into account make creating a definition possible, but several attempts have been proposed over the last 30 years. Many TRD staging models have been suggested, all of them intended to clarify the concept of TRD, but the lack of consensus represents an ongoing clinical and nosological controversy. In parallel, efforts towards a more accurate definition are aimed at proposing clear-cut criteria for clinical trials and research to evaluate specific treatment strategies and biological factors in TRD.

Treatment-resistant Depression, First Edition. Edited by Siegfried Kasper and Stuart Montgomery.
© 2013 John Wiley & Sons, Ltd. Published 2013 by John Wiley & Sons, Ltd.

Beyond a definition, efforts have been made to identify key clinical factors associated with TRD.

The purpose of this chapter is to review current available definitions and predictors of TRD originating from different fields and to discuss their usefulness in clinical practice and clinical research.

Introduction

Although TRD appears to be relatively common in clinical practice, the inconsistent way in which it has been characterized and defined remains a real problem, limiting systematic research. From a clinical point of view, TRD usually refers to an inadequate response to at least one antidepressant trial of adequate dose and duration. It is estimated that 50–60% of patients do not achieve meaningful response following antidepressant treatment (Souery *et al.*, 1999). This conception may include a variety of clinical situations, from uncomplicated failure to one course of antidepressant to multiple failures with long-term persistence of depressive symptoms despite more complex treatments. The term *treatment refractoriness* is generally used in these circumstances. While this approach corresponds to the clinical reality, it doesn't help to define TRD and to predict which depressive episode will be resistant to treatment. The huge complexity of the phenomenon and the wide variety of parameters that must be taken into account make creating a definition possible, but several attempts have been proposed over the last 30 years. Misdiagnosis ('pseudoresistance'), comorbidities, definition of treatment response, treatment duration and compliance and the number of treatment failures are among the more difficult variables which need to be integrated in any attempt to characterize or define TRD, making this a real challenge (Fornaro *et al.*, 2010).

Definitions of TRD have been considered from different perspectives and with diverse objectives. The available definitions are mostly proposed by clinicians who have in mind a direct benefit for difficult-to-treat patients. The identification of predictors for TRD shares the same concern. In parallel, efforts at providing a more accurate definition aim to propose clear-cut criteria for clinical trials and research in order to evaluate specific treatment strategies and biological factors in TRD.

The purpose of this chapter is to review current available definitions and predictors of TRD originating from different fields and to discuss their usefulness in clinical practice and clinical research.

Definition of TRD: historical perspective

The basic question that needs to be addressed in the proposed definitions remains the threshold at which we define 'treatment resistance'. This threshold is composed of multiple complex variables, foremost among which is the number of antidepressant failures. Historically, two distinct periods can be recognized in the attempt to define TRD. The poor level of attention paid to conceptual examination in the 1970s and 1980s resulted in unsystematic research and uncontrolled clinical trials, which in turn led to a degree of confusion. An analysis of the existing publications on TRD highlights a long misty period; in a review of a 10-year period of the literature covering 1985–1995, more than 15 separate definitions were proposed (Ayd, 1983; Fawcett & Kravitz, 1985; Feigner *et al.*, 1985; Fink, 1991; Links & Akiskal, 1987; McGrath *et al.*, 1987; Montgomery, 1991; Nelsen & Dunner, 1993; Roose *et al.*, 1986; Schatzberg *et al.*, 1983, 1986; Thase & Rush, 1995). This *first wave* of definitions was influential in introducing key parameters such as dose (a minimal adequate dose equivalent of 200 mg of imipramine per day), duration of treatments and number of failures, but all of the definitions differed with respect to quantification of these parameters and the hierarchy of treatment types and sequences. At this time, tricyclic antidepressants

(TCAs), monoamine oxidase inhibitors (MAOIs), lithium and electroconvulsive therapy (ECT) were among various treatments incorporated in any TRD definition, but all in different sequences and with various durations based on empirical assumptions. Feigner *et al.* (1985) proposed defining TRD as a failure to respond to either TCAs or MAOIs plus a duration of episode of at least 2 years; Links & Akiskal (1987) considered TRD a failure to respond to two TCAs, one MAOI, one ECT, one lithium and one heterocyclic trial; Fawcett & Kravitz (1987) introduced the need to apply various combinations of adequate trials of TCA, MAOI and ECT. Montgomery (1991) was the first to recommend a pragmatic approach of two antidepressant failures, anticipating the current most accepted description.

These proposals had the merit of setting the stage and emphasizing the need to propose a systematic approach in TRD. The challenge at that time was to propose clinical guidelines and treatment strategies and to initiate clinical and biological research in the field. The concept of TRD was not ready and mature enough to be considered for recognition by regulatory authorities in Europe or the USA, and no official indication for TRD was possible.

A new era opened with the emergence of more structured and practical definitions of TRD, giving priority to a descriptive approach that led to the *staging models* of TRD. Thase & Rush (1997) were the first to publish a comprehensive staging model, taking into account the number and class of treatments received in order to indicate the level of resistance. Lately, in response to the need to validate treatment strategies or specific medications in TRD, regulatory authorities in Europe and the USA have elaborated their own recommendations for use in clinical trials.

Besides the development of descriptive definitions, recent progress has been made in the identification of predictive factors for TRD. Combining such variables with the proposed definitions and staging models will certainly help to validate the concept of TRD.

TRD staging models

Several staging models have been proposed, all of them intended to clarify the concept of TRD. Although some overlap exits between these models, they mainly differ in the weight of quantitative and qualitative parameters considered. The current proposals have undoubtedly contributed to a better assessment of TRD, but the lack of consensus represents an ongoing clinical and nosological controversy (Fornaro *et al.*, 2010).

Thase and Rush model (1997)

Faced with the heterogeneity of TRD, Thase & Rush (1997) proposed applying the concept of illness classification used in oncology. Their starting point was the most common situation: the failure of a selective serotonin reuptake inhibitor (SSRI) chosen as first-line treatment. More than a simple descriptive staging model, their guideline suggested a series of sequential strategies for each stage of resistance. The recommendations were primarily based on the available publications on the management of treatment nonresponse to SSRIs. Antidepressant nonresponders are classified along a five-stage continuum according to the number and class of antidepressants that have failed to provide a response. In the final algorithm, *stage I resistance* is considered a failure of at least one adequate trial of one major class of antidepressant.

The proposed model is then built based on the assumption that switching to an alternative medication with a different mechanism of action is appropriate. A hierarchy of treatments is implied with the statement that MAOIs are more effective than TCAs, and TCAs are superior to SSRIs. The authors also discuss the use of combination and/or augmentation strategies in the most difficult-to-treat situations, after more than two failures, but do not include these strategies in the staging model.

Stage II resistance is defined as a failure of at least two adequate trials of at least two distinct classes of antidepressant. *Stage III* is stage II resistance plus failure of an adequate trial of a TCA, *stage IV* corresponds to stage III plus failure of an adequate trial of an MAOI and *stage V* is stage IV plus a course of bilateral ECT.

Trying to integrate the simple descriptive approach of the level of treatment resistance to sequential treatment strategies is useful but raises important methodological issues. It is subject to discussion or controversy over the validity of the existing data on the efficacy of the treatment strategies; this is particularly illustrated by the issue of the current and more recent data not supporting the use of antidepressants from two different classes. However, this approach is commonly used in clinical practice and is recommended in several treatment guidelines (Bauer *et al.*, 2007). The results of a recent meta-analysis comparing two switch strategies for depressed patients failing to respond to an SSRI, a second SSRI or a different class of antidepressant suggest a marginal benefit of switching from one class to another on remission rates only (Papakostas *et al.*, 2008). In contrast, other groups reported no advantage of switching classes (Bschor & Baethge, 2010; Ruhé *et al.*, 2006; Rush *et al.*, 2006).

The Thase and Rush staging model is the first attempt to integrate evidence-based data on treatment strategies and level of resistance in a comprehensive model (Thase & Rush, 1997). It represents an easy-to-use tool, providing a logical representation of the levels of resistance for clinicians. Its limitations are that dosing and duration of each sequence are not defined, and that nonresponse to two agents of different classes is assumed to be more difficult to treat than nonresponse to two agents of the same class. It may need revision based on more recent data. In addition, the staging model is limited by the implicit hierarchy of antidepressants (MAOIs > TCAs > SSRIs), for which there is no sufficient evidence in the literature.

European staging model (1999)

The Group for the Study of Resistant Depression (GSRD) developed a quantitative and sequential staging model that does not integrate treatment strategies (Souery *et al.*, 1999). Facing the complexity of definitely specifying the number of failed adequate trials needed to define resistance, the model proposes a simple continuum starting from the first antidepressant failure in the treatment of a depressive episode and continuing with all subsequent unsuccessful trials regardless of the type of treatment. The different stages correspond to the number and duration of antidepressant trials. This model is independent of the treatments used and does not imply a hierarchy of efficacy of antidepressants or treatment strategies. The controversial issue of the number and type of adequate therapeutic trials may be arbitrarily solved using this continuous-quantitative principle. The model is built on naturalistic observation of the outcomes of prescribed treatments. These operational criteria are not to be considered an absolute definition of TRD, but rather a logical instrument that can be used in clinical practice and research projects in order to classify patients based on their level of resistance.

The model proposes distinguishing between nonresponse and five levels of TRD. The starting point is the depressive episode for which lack of response is recognized and the type of drug for which resistance is observed. A single adequately treated episode of nonresponse to an antidepressant is in itself sufficient to raise the issue of resistance. Patients who do not respond to one type of adequately prescribed drug (e.g. an SSRI-resistant depressive episode) are classified as nonresponders to any antidepressant therapy. It is assumed that the dose and duration of the antidepressant trial are adequate. Following this, five levels of TRD, defined according to the number of treatments (TRD1 to TRD5), are proposed. The usual treatment duration is between 4 and 8 weeks. TRD5 corresponds to nearly 1 year of treatment containing at least five different consecutive unsuccessful antidepressants trials, while TRD1 corresponds to 1 year of treatment with one unsuccessful trial. These stages apply to acute treatments and do not consider prolonged durations of treatment resistance. An additional concept is *chronic refractory depression* (CRD), which is when a patient is treated with several antidepressants for more than 12 months with unsatisfactory response.

The advantage of the European Staging Model (ESM) is its simplicity, transposing into a continuous approach the observed outcome of adequate antidepressant trials. It can easily be used in clinical research to define the level of resistance of patients included in clinical trials, for example. It keeps open the question of any threshold in defining TRD based on the number of failed trials. However, it may be considered incomplete since it does not consider the weight of treatment strategies such as augmentation, combination or ECT. It may be misleading in distinguishing between nonresponse and resistance, with resistance being viewed as a lack of response after two failures. Nonresponse should be considered the first level of TRD.

Massachusetts general hospital staging model (2003)

The Massachusetts General Hospital staging method (MGH-S) is also primarily a quantitative approach, generating a continuous score that represents the degree of resistance (Fava, 2003). Three categories of score are proposed, integrating the number of trials and types of treatment strategy.

In category 1, nonresponse to each in a sequence of adequate (at least 6 weeks of an adequate dosage of an antidepressant) antidepressant trials increases the score by 1 point. While the labelling of each stage uses scores instead of TRD categories (TRD1 to TRD5), this approach is similar to that of the ESM. There is no limit to the number of failed trials, which are not considered from a longitudinal perspective. The MGH-S differs in considering augmentation and optimization strategies in the degree of resistance. ECT is also included in the model.

In category 2, the global score of resistance is increased by 0.5 points per trial when an optimization or augmentation strategy is used: optimization of dose and duration, and augmentation or combination of each trial. The MHG-S was developed together with the Massachusetts General Hospital or Antidepressant Treatment Response Questionnaire, a useful tool for collecting reliable data on previous treatments.

In category 3, the score is further increased by 3 points if ECT is applied.

The MHG-S makes no distinction and builds no hierarchy based on antidepressant mechanism of action. In category 1, any adequate trial with any antidepressant will increase the score. In category 2, augmentation, combination, dosage and duration optimization are equally weighted. A qualitative component is incorporated in the apparent quantitative approach in category 2 and 3 scores, where scores of 0.5 and 3 are artificially attributed to optimization and ECT, respectively. The MHG-S was examined for reliability in predicting nonremission in a retrospective analysis, and demonstrated greater ability than the Thase and Rush method (Petersen *et al.*, 2005).

Maudsley staging model (2009)

Most of the existing staging models rely on treatment response and number of medications as key criteria by which to define TRD. While the lack of efficacy of a prescribed antidepressant represents a core element of treatment resistance, many other factors related to the depressive episode need to be considered. This multidimensional approach has clearly been neglected in previously proposed definitions of TRD.

Parker *et al.* (2005) have identified a set of key elements related to mood states unresponsive to treatments that are not considered in most TRD definitions. These proposed 'paradigm failures' include failure to diagnose and manage bipolar disorder, failure to diagnose and manage psychotic depression, failure to diagnose and manage melancholic depression, diagnosis and/or management of a nonmelancholic condition as if it were melancholic depression, misdiagnosis of secondary depression and failure to identify organic determinants. Failure to adequately assess the severity or type of depression and failure to identify organic determinants are the main causes of misclassification of depressive episodes not responding to treatment.

Beyond the treatment-outcome parameter, the multidimensional nature of TRD has been considered in developing the Maudsley staging model (MSM) (Fekadu *et al.*, 2009). Treatment resistance is viewed as a continuum produced and maintained by various dimensional factors. The severity and duration of a depressive illness are incorporated in this staging model of TRD, while the number of treatments sequentially failing to produce improvement remains a key parameter in the level of resistance. Between- and within-class switching and type of treatment are not considered in the MSM.

Three sets of parameters/dimensions are integrated in the model: *duration*, *symptoms severity* and *treatment failures*:

- The *duration* of the presenting episode is classified into three categories: acute (1 year or less), subacute (between 1 and 2 years) and chronic (longer than 2 years). The duration of the episode is specified irrespective of treatment experience and scored from 1 to 3.
- The *severity dimension* is based on the International Statistical Classification of Diseases and Related Health Problems, 10th revision (ICD-10) classification of syndromal depression (mild, moderate, severe without psychosis and severe with psychosis). Subsyndromal depression is also included in the symptom-severity variable. Severity is scored from 1 to 5.
- In the *treatment failures* parameter, five levels are proposed (from level 1: 1–2 medications to level 5: >10 medications). Treatment failures also includes augmentation used or not (score 0 or 1) and ECT used or not (score 0 or 1). The maximal score for treatment failures is 7.

The global TRD score should be between 3 and 15. Staging of resistance can be expressed in three categories: mild (scores 3–6), moderate (scores 7–10) and severe (scores 11–15). The principal added value of the model consists in the possibility of emphasizing in each case the most important factors of the presenting episode contributing to resistance to treatment. As stated by the authors, the model does not include psychosocial stressors or functional impairment.

The MSM was validated through prospective fellow-up study and showed significant association with persistence of depressive disorder (Fekadu *et al.*, 2009).

Definition of TRD in clinical trials

A growing number of studies looking at the efficacy of therapeutic interventions in TRD have been published in the last decade. A systematic review of randomized clinical trials of antidepressant use in TRD highlights the variability in the ascertainment of TRD (Berlim & Turecki, 2007). Among the 47 randomized clinical trials analysed, the majority did not use systematic methods to collect data on previous treatments at baseline. The number of failed trials required to define TRD varied considerably across studies, ranging from nonresponse to one treatment to nonresponse to two or more antidepressants. In eight studies, this information was not available. The other randomized studies used at least six different definitions of TRD based on the number of previous antidepressant failures and the need to have antidepressants with different mechanisms of action. The available studies also differed in diagnostic evaluation of the depressive episode, treatment outcome, treatment duration, treatment dosage and compliance.

Lack of consensus on these issues clearly limits the interpretation of findings and their translation to clinical practice in terms of treatment efficacy in the management of TRD (Berlim & Turecki, 2007).

In Europe, no specific treatments have been approved for TRD, and the available staging models have been considered of limited value in the regulatory setting. The European Medicines Agency (EMA) guideline on the clinical investigation of medicinal products in the treatment of depression (European Agency for the Evaluation of Medicinal Products, 2002) considers monotherapy in patients with TRD a separate claim and proposes a clinical trial design and definition for TRD. TRD is considered *when treatment with at least two different antidepressant agents prescribed in adequate dosages for adequate duration and with adequate affirmation of treatment adherence showed lack of clinically meaningful improvement.* This pragmatic definition differs from the complex available staging models but is mainly intended to be used within clinical trials as a reference by which to characterize patients based on the number and type of previous treatments.

This EMA definition differs from that of previous versions, where two products of different pharmacological classes were requested. This important revision is in line with the most recent data, showing no advantage in favour of switching to a different class of antidepressant (Bschor & Baethge, 2010; Papakostas *et al.*, 2008; Ruhé *et al.*, 2006; Rush *et al.*, 2006; Souery *et al.*, 2011a, 2011b).

A compound with substantiated general major depression indication needs at least one additional trial using this definition in order to support extension of the indication to TRD. The proposed study design requires that at least one treatment failure should be prospectively shown. Patients are included in clinical trials based on retrospective assessment of treatment failure to at least one adequate antidepressant. Following this, prospective confirmation of treatment failure to the next antidepressant is needed. Patients are then randomized to receive the investigated medication or the active comparator.

The EMA guidelines exclude the use of augmentation strategy in TRD. Augmentation is considered a separate indication for partial responders. Patients with TRD (who show no clinically meaningful change from baseline as result of treatment) are not suitable candidates for augmentation as there is no response to augment.

Clinical characteristics and predictors of TRD

Beyond the definition, the identification of factors associated with TRD remains unclear. Numerous studies have been performed with the aim of identifying predictive factors of treatment response to antidepressants, but the heterogeneity in the definitions or criteria used for treatment response and the small sample sizes limit replication and prevent definitive conclusions (Nierenberg, 2003). Misdiagnosis, suboptimal treatment and duration of illness remain among the more frequently encountered problems. Despite these difficulties in defining TRD, there is evidence that both poor response and persistent depression can be predicted by specific variables.

Genetic determinants of treatment response to antidepressants have been investigated but currently their role remains limited in clinical practice. The most significant and replicated findings concern the gene encoding for the serotonin transporter (SERT), particularly its functional polymorphism located in the SERT promoter region (SERTPR) (Serretti *et al.*, 2009).

Outcome studies of nonresponse to antidepressants have been able to recognize a number of demographic and clinical characteristics. It should be noted that these variables are based on the results of uncontrolled, retrospective or long-term prospective studies of chronic depression and may include a significant proportion of pseudoresistant cases.

At the clinical level, frequent issues associated with nonresponse remain severity, chronicity and comorbid symptoms. Comorbid psychiatric disorders include substance abuse or dependence, personality disorders, eating disorders, obsessive–compulsive disorders and panic or generalized anxiety disorders (Hirschfeld *et al.*, 1988; Maser & Cloninger, 1990). In treatment failure, a thorough evaluation of these conditions should always be considered. It has been observed that in depression, concomitant personality disorders reduce the efficacy of antidepressant treatments and may contribute towards treatment resistance (Black *et al.*, 1988; Pfohl *et al.*, 1984; Shea *et al.*, 1990, 1992). It is not clear, therefore, whether the observed 'treatment resistance' relates to the depressive state or the comorbid personality disorder (Thase, 1996). Older age and female sex appear to be associated with a higher risk of nonresponse to antidepressant treatment (Keller *et al.*, 1986; Paykel *et al.*, 1973). The illness characteristics that have been frequently associated with poor response are unipolar illness, psychotic depression, neurotic premorbid personality, familial predisposition to affective disorders, multiple loss events and a low socioeconomic level (Burrows *et al.*, 1994; Scott, 1995; Scott & Eccleston, 1991). A range of concurrent medical conditions may also contribute to TRD; results from several studies have shown that thyroid dysfunction may be associated with it (Gold *et al.*, 1981; Hatterrer & Gorman, 1990; Howland, 1993). Other medical conditions have been implicated as organic causes of depression and require documentation and exclusion in TRD (Gruber *et al.*, 1996). They should be labelled as mood disorder due to a general medical condition. Examples of such conditions are Cushing's syndrome, Parkinson's disease, neurological neoplasms, pancreatic carcinoma, connective-tissue disorders, vitamin deficiencies and certain viral infections. Several types of medication, such as beta-blockers, immunosuppressants, steroids and sedatives, may also precipitate or contribute to chronic depression and adversely affect remission and response.

These factors seem to influence treatment response to antidepressant therapy, but more research is needed to clarify their weight in the variability of treatment response (Serretti *et al.*, 2009).

The investigation of clinical factors associated with TRD has mostly been conducted through studies looking at nonresponse to a single antidepressant treatment, without taking into account multiple treatment failures. Very few studies have been conducted on clinical features associated with failure to at least two consecutive antidepressant trials. The GSRD conducted the largest study on specific clinical and demographic factors associated with major depressive disorder (MDD) in patients who failed to reach response or remission after at least two consecutive adequate antidepressants (Souery *et al.*, 2007). Demographic, diagnostic and treatment outcome data were available for a total of 955 patients who met criteria for a major depressive episode and had received at least 4 weeks' adequate antidepressant treatment at optimal dose. Among these patients, 702 received at least two consecutive antidepressant trials for their current or last episode and were thus considered for the analysis. A total of 229 reached a HAM-D-17 score < 17 after the initial antidepressant and 117 had a score < 17 after a second

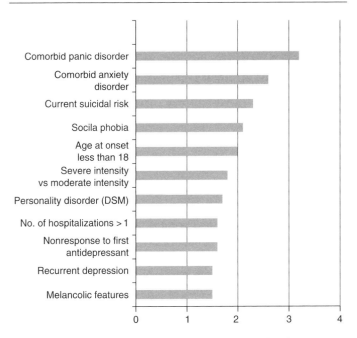

Figure 1.1   Odds ratios for clinical factors associated with treatment-resistant depression (TRD) in the European multicentre study performed by the Group for the Study of Resistant Depression (GSRD) (Souery *et al.*, 2007). Variables with p values < 0.05

consecutive antidepressant trial following failure of the initial trial. These 346 patients were considered 'nonresistant'. The remaining 356 patients were considered 'resistant' as their HAM-D-17 score remained greater than or equal to 17 after two consecutive adequate antidepressant trials.

A Cox logistic regression model was applied in the search for factors associated with resistance. The clinical factors significantly associated (p values < 0.05) with TRD are shown in Figure 1.1, ranked by odds ratios. Given the likelihood that several clinical variables are correlated, a stepwise Cox regression model was used to independently test the factors associated with TRD in the first step. Four variables emerged as being independently correlated to TRD: comorbid anxiety disorder, current suicidal risk, melancholic features and nonresponse to first antidepressant lifetime.

Although the retrospective assessment represents a limitation of the study, the findings provide a set of relevant clinical variables associated with treatment resistance, defined as nonresponse to two consecutive antidepressant trials, regardless of mechanism of action.

Conclusions

The definition of TRD has acquired a certain maturity thanks to the staging models published over the last 15 years. These models include most of the key parameters needed to conceptualize TRD and allow for a better characterization of patients. We have to admit that these efforts towards a better definition of TRD exist with insufficient dialogue and with very few exchanges between the various research centres involved. It will be necessary to create an international network of reflection on the subject in order to allow us to reach a consensus. This is important not only for the clinical approach but also and especially for research on treatment strategies and the biology of TRD. It is also essential to move the interests and views of clinicians closer to those of regulatory authorities.

References

Ayd, F. J. (1983) Treatment resistant depression. *Int. Drug Ther. Newsletter*, **18**, 25–27.

Bauer, M., Bschor, T., Pfennig, A. *et al*. (2007) World Federation of Societies of Biological Psychiatry (WFSBP) guidelines for biological treatment of unipolar depressive disorders in primary care. *World J. Biol. Psychiatry*, **8**(2), 67–104.

Berlim, M. T. & Turecki, G. (2007) What is the meaning of treatment resistant/refractory major depression (TRD)? A systematic review of current randomized trials. *Eur. Neuropsychopharmacol.*, **17**(11), 696–707.

Black, D. W., Bell, S., Hubert, J. *et al*. (1988) The importance of axis II in patients with major depression. *J. Affect. Disord*., **14**, 115–122.

Bschor, T. & Baethge, C. (2010) No evidence for switching the anti-depressant: systematic review and meta-analysis of RCTs of a common therapeutic strategy. *Acta Psychiatr. Scand*., **121**, 174–179.

Burrows, G. D., Norman, T. R. & Judd, F. K. (1994) Definition and differential diagnosis of treatment-resistant depression. *Intern. Clin. Psychopharm.*, **9**(2), 5–10.

European Agency for the Evaluation of Medicinal Products (2002) Evaluation of Medicines for Human Use. Note for Guidance on Clinical Investigation of Medicinal Products in the Treatment of Depression. European Agency for the Evaluation of Medicinal Products, London, UK. April 25, 2002. CPMP/EWP/518/97, Rev.1. Available at: http://www.emea.europa.eu/pdfs/human/ewp/051897en.pdf, last accessed November 9, 2012.

Fava, M. (2003) Diagnosis and definition of treatment resistant depression. *Biol. Psychiatry*, **53**, 649–659.

Fawcett, J. & Kravitz, H. M. (1985) Treatment refractory depression, in *Common Treatment Problems in Depression* (ed. A. F. Schatzberg), American Psychiatric Press, Washington, DC, USA.

Feigner, J. P., Herbstein, J. & Damlouji, N. (1985) Combined MAOI, TCA, and direct stimulant therapy of treatment-resistant depres-sion. *J. Clin. Psychiatry*, **46**, 206–209.

Fekadu, A., Wooderson, S. C., Markopoulou, K. *et al*. (2009) Maudsley Staging Method for treatment-resistant depression: prediction of longer-term outcome and persistence of symptoms. *J. Clin. Psychiatry*, **70**(7), 952–957.

Fink, M. (1991) A trial of ECT is essential before a diagnosis of refractory depression is made, in *Advances in Neuropsychiatry and Psychopharmacology: Vol. 2. Refractory Depression* (ed. J. D. Amsterdam), Raven Press, New York, NY, USA, pp. 87–92.

Fornaro, M. & Giosuè, P. (2010) Current nosology of treatment resist-ant depression: a controversy resistant to revision. *Clin. Pract. Epidemiol. Ment. Health*, **4**(6), 20–24.

Gold, M. S., Pottash, A. L. C. & Extein, I. (1981) Hypothyroidism and depression. *JAMA*, **245**, 1919–1922.

Gruber, A. J., Hudson, J. I. & Pope, H. G. (1996) The management of treatment-resistant depression in disorders on the interface of psychiatry and medicine. *Psychiatr. Clin. North Am*., **19**(2), 351–361.

Hatterrer, J. A. & Gorman, J. M. (1990) Thyroid function in refractory depression, in *Treatment Strategies for Refractory Depression* (ed. S. P. Roose & A. H. Glassman), American Psychiatry Press, Washington, DC, USA, pp. 171–191.

Hirschfeld, R. M. A., Kosier, T., Keller, M. B. *et al*. (1988) The influence of alcoholism on the course of depression. *J. Affect. Disord.*, **16**, 151–158.

Howland, R. H. (1993) Thyroid dysfunction in refractory depression: implications for pathophysiology and treatment. *J. Clin. Psychiatry*, **54**, 47–54.

Keller, M. B., Lavori, P. W., Rice, J. *et al*. (1986) The persistent risk of chronicity in recurrent episodes of non-bipolar depressive disorder: a prospective follow-up. *Am. J. Psychiatry*, **143**, 24–28.

Links, P. S. & Akiskal, H. S. (1987) Chronic and intractable depressions: terminology, classification, and description of subtypes, in *Treating Resistant Depression* (ed. J. Zohar & R. H. Belmaker), PMA Publishing, New York, NY, USA, pp. 1–22.

Maser, J. D. & Cloninger, R. C. (1990) *Comorbidity of Mood and Anxiety Disorders*, American Psychiatric Press, Washington, DC, USA.

McGrath, P. J., Stewart, J. W., Harrison, W. *et al*. (1987) Treatment of refractory depression with a monoamine oxidase inhibitor antidepressant. *Psychopharmacol. Bulletin*, **23**, 169–173.

Montgomery, S. A. (1991) Selectivity of antidepressants and resistant depression, in *Advances in Neuropsychiatry and Psychopharmacology: Vol. 2. Refractory Depression* (ed. J. D. Amsterdam), Raven Press, New York, NY, USA, pp. 93–104.

Nelsen, M. R. & Dunner, D. L. (1993) Treatment resistance in unipolar depression and other disorders. *Psychiatr. Clin. North Am.*, **16**(3), 541–566.

Nierenberg, A. A. (2003) Predictors of response to antidepressants general principles and clinical implications. *Psychiatr. Clin. North Am.*, **26**(2), 345–352.

Papakostas, G. I., Fava, M. & Thase, M. E. (2008) Treatment of SSRI-resistant depression: a meta-analysis comparing within- versus across-class switches. *Biol. Psychiatry*, **63**, 699–704.

Parker, G. B., Malhi, G. S., Crawford, J. G. & Thase, M. E. (2005) Identifying 'paradigm failures' contributing to treatment-resistant depression. *J. Affect. Disord.*, **87**(2–3), 185–191.

Paykel, E. S., Prussoff, B., Klerman, G. L. *et al*. (1973) A clinical response to amitriptyline among depressed women. *J. Nerv. Ment. Dis.*, **156**, 149–165.

Petersen, T., Papakostas, G. I., Posternak, M. A. *et al*. (2005) Empirical testing of two models for staging antidepressant treatment resistance. *J. Clin. Psychopharmacol.*, **25**(4), 336–341.

Pfohl, B., Stangl, D. & Zimmerman, M. (1984) The implications of DSM-III personality disorders for patients with major depression. *J. Affect. Disord.*, **7**, 309–318.

Roose, S. P., Glassman, A. H., Walsh, T. & Woodring, S. (1986) Tricyclic non-responders: phenomology and treatment. *Am. J. Psychiatry*, **143**, 345–348.

Ruhé, H. G., Huyser, J., Swinkels, J. A. & Schene, A. H. (2006) Switching antidepressants after a first selective serotonin reuptake inhibitor in major depressive disorder: a systematic review. *J. Clin. Psychiatry*, **67**(12), 1836–1855.

Rush, A. J., Trivedi, M. H., Wisniewski, S. R. *et al*. (2006) Acute and longer-term outcomes in depressed outpatients requiring one or several treatment steps: a STAR*D report. *Am. J. Psychiatry*, **163**(11), 1905–1917.

Schatzberg, A. F., Cole, J. O., Cohen, B. M. *et al*. (1983) Survey of depressed patients who have failed to respond to treatment, in *The Affective Disorders* (ed. J. M. Davis & J. W. Maas), American Psychiatric Press, Washington, DC, USA, pp. 73–85.

Schatzberg, A. F., Cole, J. O., Elliott, G. R. (1986) Recent views on treatment resistant depression, in *Psychosocial Aspects of Non-response to Antidepressant Drugs* (ed. U. Halbreich & S. S. Feinberg), American Psychiatric Press, Washington, DC, USA, pp. 95–109.

Scott, J. (1995) Predictors of non-response to antidepressants, in *Refractory Depression: Current Strategies and Future Directions* (ed. W. A. Nolen, J. Zohar, S. P. Roose & J. D. Amsterdam), John Wiley & Sons, London.

Scott, J. & Eccleston, D. (1991) Prediction, treatment and prognosis of major depression. *Int. Clin. Psychopharmacol.*, **6**(Suppl. 1), 41–49.

Serretti, A., Chiesa, A., Calati, R. *et al*. (2009) Common genetic, clinical, demographic and psychosocial predictors of response to pharmacotherapy in mood and anxiety disorders. *Int. Clin. Psychopharmacol.*, **24**(1), 1–18.

Shea, M. T., Pilkonis, P. A., Beckham, E. *et al*. (1990) Personality disorder and treatment outcome in the NIMH treatment of depression collaborative research program. *Am. J. Psychiatry*, **147**, 711–718.

Shea, M. T., Wuidiger, T. A. & Klein, M. H. (1992) Comorbidity of personality disorders and depression: implications for treatment. *J. Cons. Clin. Psychol.*, **60**, 857–868.

Souery, D., Amsterdam, J., de Montigny, C. *et al.* (1999) Treatment resistant depression: methodological overview and operational criteria. *Eur. Neuropsychopharmacol.*, **9**(1–2), 83–91.

Souery, D., Oswald, P., Massat, I. *et al.* (2007) Clinical factors associated with treatment resistance in major depression: results from a European multicenter study. *J. Clin. Psychiatry*, **68**(7), 1062–1070.

Souery, D., Serretti, A., Calati, A. *et al.* (2011a) Citalopram versus desipramine in treatment resistant depression: effect of continuation or switching strategies: a randomized open study. *World J. Biol. Psychiatry*, **12**(5), 364–375.

Souery, D., Serretti, A., Calati, R. *et al.* (2011b) Switching antidepressant class does not improve response or remission in treatment-resistant depression. *J. Clin. Psychopharmacol.*, **31**(4), 512–516.

Thase, M. E. (1996) The role of axis II comorbidity in the management of patients with treatment-resistant depression. *Psychiatr. Clin. North Am.*, **19**(2), 287–292.

Thase, M. E. & Rush, A. J. (1995) Treatment-resistant depression, in *Psychopharmacology: The Fourth Generation of Progress* (ed. F. E. Bloom & D. J. Kupfer), Raven Press, New York, NY, USA.

Thase, M. E. & Rush, A. J. (1997) When at first you don't succeed: sequential strategies for antidepressant nonresponders. *J. Clin. Psychiatry*, **58**(Suppl. 13), 23–29.

CHAPTER 2

Treatment-resistant Depression: A Separate Disorder – A New Approach

**Hans-Jürgen Möller, Florian Seemüller
and Rebecca Schennach**
*Department of Psychiatry and Psychotherapy,
Ludwig Maximilians University, Munich, Germany*

Ramesh K. Gupta
*Consultation and Liaison Psychiatry Unit,
The Canberra Hospital, Canberra, Australia*

Summary

Psychiatric diagnostic terminology is considered the weak component of modern research. The use of the terms 'treatment-resistant depression' (TRD), 'refractory depression', 'difficult-to-treat depression' and 'chronic depression' demonstrates such weakness. There is no body of literature that refers to any international agreement on the operational definition of TRD or its

Treatment-resistant Depression, First Edition. Edited by Siegfried Kasper
and Stuart Montgomery.
© 2013 John Wiley & Sons, Ltd. Published 2013 by John Wiley & Sons, Ltd.

predispositions, symptoms, physical signs, clinical investigations or treatment outcomes. Thus far, no phenotypic identity for patients with TRD has been defined. The serious clinical ramifications of this condition warrant a more conventional medical identity, concern and approach.

In this chapter, we briefly summarize the development of various TRD concepts and present data from a large inpatient cohort using the multidimensional Maudsley staging method (MSM) to fortify the view that patients with TRD should be given more prominence. We propose that a new prefix should be taken from medicine to name TRD 'malignant' or 'pernicious' or 'virulent' depression instead. In support of our suggestion, we also describe the inclusion criteria for this category of patients. Given the nature of new developments in therapeutic modalities for TRD patients, such as ketamine therapy and deep-brain stimulation (DBS), it is opportune to open the debate over new terminology for TRD. This exercise may be of value in research, in phenotypic identity, in ethical and in research funding considerations in this field.

Introduction

It is arguable whether major depression in its current form will remain unaltered as a diagnostic category, as there is a body of opinion seeking modifications to the operational criteria in the Diagnostic and Statistical Manual of Mental Disorders, 4th edition (DSM-IV) (Gupta, 2009; Parker, 2005, 2008; Zimmerman, 2006). In the meantime, a large number of patients continue to be categorized as suffering from a definite and recognized sequel to the diagnosis of major depression under the varied rubrics of TRD, 'difficult-to-treat depression', 'treatment-refractory depression', 'residual depression' and the overlapping term, 'chronic depression'. During the last 5 years, more than 2600 articles reviewing TRD, refractory depression, difficult-to-treat depression and lengthy depression have appeared in the scientific journals on PubMed. Most of these articles are focussed on treatment strategies for patients described by these terms. There is no body of literature that refers to any international agreement on the operational definition of TRD, or its predispositions, symptoms, physical signs, clinical investigations and treatment outcomes. Some authors have shown their discontent with the various terms listed here in the context of their own research (Berlim & Turecki, 2007; Parker, 2005; Sourey, 2007).

There is a need to know what becomes of these patients once they have been identified as having TRD or as they are treated with various antidepressant therapies. Do they now fall into a cluster/syndrome distinct to that they were in when their illness started? What clinical signs and symptoms and pathophysiological changes (if any) do they have? Could these patients further our understanding and advance research beyond sequential therapies? This paper reviews this topic and makes proposals with these considerations in mind.

Historical background

Robins & Guze (1972) reviewed 20 longitudinal studies of affective disorders and found that a chronic course would apply to 1–28% of patients suffering from depressive illness. A naturalistic follow-up component of the American National Institute of Mental Health Collaborative Psychobiology Program observed that 21% of patients had not recovered 2 years after an episode of major depression and 12% had not recovered after 5 years (Keller *et al.*, 1984). Furthermore, the cumulative risk that an individual who had suffered from primary or secondary depression would eventually develop a chronic illness was about 30% (Keller, 1985). Kielholz (1986) concluded that 15–20% of depressed patients required hospitalization, most of them because their depression was resistant to antidepressant therapy. Kiloh *et al.* (1988) followed 133 patients who were diagnosed with primary depressive illness for a 15-year period and noted that at the end of their study, 7% had committed suicide, 12% remained incapacitated and only 20% were leading normal lives. Scott (1988) proposed that the most appropriate term by which to describe unremitting depressions of more than 2 years' duration was 'chronic depression'. It might be that chronicity is a natural analogue of TRD and that failure to remit spontaneously over 2–5 years of depression is comparable to a failure to respond to a 6–9 month course of sequential therapies.

From a prospective 12-year follow-up study, Judd *et al.* (1988) concluded that the long-term course of unipolar major depressive illness was dominated by prolonged symptomatic chronicity, with 15% of patients suffering symptoms with full syndrome intensity, and another 43% suffering symptoms with subsyndrome severity. Thase & Rush (1995) reviewed a much larger body of literature and reached a similar conclusion. In a 25-year longitudinal comparison study of the outcome of depression, Brodaty *et al.* (2001) found that only 12% of patients remained continuously well; following antidepressant treatments, 50–60% of patients did not achieve adequate response (Fava, 2003; Kupfer, 2003). Another study showed that one-third of patients failed to have sufficient symptom improvement despite adequate treatment (Klein *et al.*, 2004). Kennedy and colleagues (2004) interviewed a cohort who had suffered acute depression 8–11 years after the initial acute episode and found that 13% were still suffering depression at the full syndrome level and another 20% at the subsyndromal level. A 9-month longitudinal investigation of major depression outcome studies in primary care, conducted across six different countries, showed a complete remission in only 25–48% of patients, with the remainder continuing to have symptoms (Fleck *et al.*, 2005). The wide variation in the treatment outcome in these studies is probably attributable to differing patient populations, diagnostic criteria for depression, assessment methods and frequencies of follow-up. Depressed patients are twice as likely to be treated these days as they were, say, 20 years ago, and the overall outcome for individually treated patients with antidepressant therapies has improved considerably (Möller, 2009). However, depression among patients aged 55 years or more in primary care continues to have a poor prognosis (Licht-Strunk, 2009), and misidentifications of even a modest prevalence of depression in primary care outnumber missed cases (Mitchell, 2009).

Current TRD concepts and their limitations

Burrows and colleagues (1994) provided the first pragmatic definition for TRD, as 'a failure to respond adequately to two successive courses of monotherapy with pharmacologically different antidepressants, given in adequate dose for sufficient time'. Phillips & Nierenberg (1994) used the terms 'treatment-refractory depression' and 'TRD' interchangeably.

Thase & Rush (1997) recommended a five-stage strategy ranging from lesser to greater degrees of treatment resistance in depression using sequential therapies. This concept remained incomplete, as it did not provide for assessments of a patient's medical status, included no comment on pathogenesis and showed no ability to differentiate the clinical symptoms on a continuum of neurotic and psychotic dimension. Furthermore, there were no evidence-based data provided in support of the recommended hierarchy of treatments and the augmentation regimens.

The quantitative Massachusetts General Hospital staging method (MGH-S) (Fava, 2003) mainly relies on the number of antidepressant medicines used to estimate the degree of resistance. Treatment vigour, treatment augmentations and failure of electroconvulsive therapy (ECT) are given weight, without adequate probing and the reason behind such weight being provided. The MGH-S model suffers from a problem in that it allows as many attempts at treatment as there are medicines available on the market, thus making it less efficient and specific.

Petersen and colleagues (2005) tested both the Thase and Rush and the MGH-S models and found that the hierarchical manner in which treatment resistance has been measured may not be strongly supported by empirical evidence. The European

Union's Committee for Proprietary Medicinal Products (Sourey *et al.*, 1999) guidelines take the view that TRD is consecutive treatments with two products of different classes, used for a sufficient length of time at an adequate dose, that fail to induce an acceptable effect. In this method, it is not clear how the differential between the efficacies of various antidepressants has been worked out.

The model proposed by Mahli *et al.* (2005) is based on the dichotomy of depression subtypes and the dimension of severity.

Parker and colleagues (2005) studied 164 patients with severe and difficult-to-treat depression referred to a tertiary centre for treatment. These authors drew attention to paradigm failures contributing to TRD, including misdiagnosis, inadequate clinical investigation, missing a diagnosis of bipolar illness and of melancholic depression, and failure therefore to provide illness- or diagnosis-specific appropriate treatment, as all depressions may not be the same. The findings of Sourey *et al.* (2006) provide a set of 11 relevant clinical variables associated with treatment resistance with comorbid anxiety disorder as the most powerful clinical factor associated with TRD.

More recently, Fekadu *et al.* (2009) proposed their multidimensional Maudsley staging method (MSM). This method quantifies treatment resistance based on a point-scoring system for the duration of illness, symptom severity, treatment failures and whether augmentation and ECT have been attempted or not. It divides treatment resistance into mild, moderate and severe categories, with cutoff scores (Table 2.1). In a further paper, Fekadu *et al.* (2009) demonstrated that the MSM has a reasonable predictive validity regarding the long-term course and outcome of illness, especially the persistence of depressive episodes (Table 2.2). The authors modelled a data analysis adjusting different variables such as gender, marital status, duration of hospital admission and the duration follow-up in coming to an odds ratio. In model 2, this would indicate a nearly twofold risk (1.89) for a new episode. So far, in spite of some limitations, this is one of the most precise instruments by which to assess TRD, as it relies on multiple dimensions.

Table 2.1 Mausdley staging parameters and suggested scoring conventions. Reproduced from Fekadu et al., The Maudsley Staging Method for Treatment-Resistant Depression: Prediction of Longer-Term Outcome and Persistence of Symptoms. *The Journal of Clinical Psychiatry*, 70(7), 952–957, 2009. Copyright 2009

Parameter/dimension	Parameter specification	Score
Duration	Acute (≤12 months)	1
	Subacute (13–24 months)	2
	Chronic (>24 months)	3
Symptom severity (at baseline)	Subsyndromal	1
	Syndromal	
	Mild	2
	Moderate	3
	Severe without psychosis	4
	Severe with psychosis	5
Treatment failures (antidepressants)	Level 1: 1–2 medications	1
	Level 2: 3–4 medications	2
	Level 3: 5–6 medications	3
	Level 4: 7–10 medications	4
	Level 5: >10 medications	5
Augmentation	Not used	0
	Used	1
ECT	Not used	0
	Used	1
TOTAL		15

Kräupl Taylor (1971) suggested that for a patient to be labelled as suffering from TRD, they must have the experience of being unwell to the extent that they would complain about it, or arouse therapeutic concern in their therapist. Such an experience must deviate from the normal in a statistically significant way. Equating an illness with a 'complaint' in such a way would entitle a patient to be the sole arbiter of whether they are ill. What if someone had no insight into their own illness, or had no therapist, or did not complain? Some individuals who should

Table 2.2 Prediction of clinical and functional status at the end of follow-up using the Maudsley staging method (MSM), adjusted for relevant clinical and sociodemographic factors. Reproduced from Fekadu *et al.*, A multidimensional tool to quantify treatment resistance in depression: the Maudsley Staging Method. *The Journal of Clinical Psychiatry,* 70(2), 177–184, 2009. Copyright 2009

Outcome/model[a]	Odds ratio	95% CI	p value
In an episode at time of final interview			
MSM score (crude)	1.46	1.06–2.02	.021
Model 1[b]	1.71	1.11–2.63	.015
Model 2[c]	1.89	1.17–3.05	.010
Functional impairment at follow-up			
MSM score (crude)	1.57	1.14–2.15	.005
Model 1[d]	1.48	1.06–2.06	.021
Model 2[c]	1.55	1.08–2.22	.017

[a]All models used at the binary logistic regression method.
[b]Adjusted for age and years of education.
[c]Additionally adjusted for sex, marital status, duration of hospital admission and duration of follow-up.
[d]Adjusted for years of education.

complain do not, and others who complain repeatedly do not seem to have adequate reasons for doing so. Equating an illness with 'therapeutic concern' also implies that no one can be ill until they have been recognized as such (Kendal, 1975). It is in criteria of this kind that the current concepts of TRD are embedded, where patients complain and psychiatrists provide treatment (this type of approach has attracted serious criticism of psychiatry in the past (Laing, 1967)). Thus the current concept of TRD can be reduced to what people complain about or what doctors treat, or a combination of the two. Such a concept is fragile at its boundaries, as it expands or contracts with changes in medicosocial attitudes towards therapeutic optimisms. It is also at the mercy of idiosyncratic decisions taken by doctors or patients and is open to pharmaceutical manipulations.

We therefore adopted the MSM, for its multidimensional and quantitative nature, to study a large sample of depressed inpatients in order to further analyse the characteristics of patients with different levels of TRD. We examined a naturalistic multicentre cohort of 644 patients who received or continued to receive treatment at the various university and district psychiatric clinics in Germany for TRD. We were able to identify 24 patients who scored 11 or more (one patient with a score of 13, two with a score of 12 and the rest with a score of 11) and thus satisfied the criteria for severe TRD according to the MSM. A total of 410 patients were between the scores of 7 and 10, being in the moderate resistant group, and 115 were below a score of 7, with minimal treatment resistance. We compared the average Hamilton scores of patients with mild (mean 22.67, SD 5.69) and severe (mean 28.38, SD 6.58) TRD, and found the difference between them achieved a significance of p value 0.0001. We discovered sadness of mood, guilt, hopelessness with suicidal preoccupation, early morning insomnia, loss of interest with impaired functioning and psychic anxiety as the dominant clinical items of significance among our cohort. These are represented on the Hamilton depression rating scale as items 1, 2, 3, 6, 7, 8, 10 progressively. Among the 24 cases of severe TRD patients, we were able to identify six as having melancholic features, as defined by DSM-IV criteria. Since our intention is to define a true phenotype for severe TRD, we will leave the six melancholic TRD standing separately, as melancholia is considered to have its own identity.

We are now able to clearly identify the clinical characteristics of severe TRD patients. These patients have sadness of mood, hopelessness, sleep disturbance, loss of interest, impaired functioning and psychic anxiety, and these characteristics, with an MSM score of 11 or more, put these patients in a category of their own. We propose to define such a separate category in the remaining part of this chapter.

Towards a new definition and nosology

The concept of disease as a syndrome – a constellation of related symptoms with a characteristic prognosis – originated with

Sydenham in the 17th century. Prior to this, the ancient-world physicians recognized symptoms such as fever, joint pains, heart burns and headaches as separate diseases to be diagnosed and treated individually. In the latter half of the 18th century, Morgagni and Bichat advanced clinical observation at the bedside to correlate these symptoms with a characteristic morbid anatomy through post-mortem dissection of the body. The development of powerful microscopes in the middle of the 19th century made it possible for individual cells to be studied for the first time, and the consequent detection of cellular pathology led Virchow and other pathologists to assume that cellular derangements were the basis of all disease. The discovery of bacteria by Koch and Pasteur further helped explain infection as the basis of some major illnesses. Thus we see how medicine in the 19th century developed syndrome identities and, where possible, aetiopathic clusters. These eventually helped us recognize the true nature of illnesses.

While psychiatry continues to have difficulty in establishing such clear aetiopathic clusters, it is foreseeable that this could happen in the near future. The role of multifactor pathogenesis of major depressions, its variable course in some cases leading to treatment resistance, is being increasingly understood. The adaptation to chronic stress and its influence on the hypothalamic–pituitary–adrenal (HPA) axis (Thompson, 2008), the role of the immune system and the induction of gene expression are examples of such advances in our understanding. Therefore, now more than ever, it is necessary to define phenotypes that are representative of true syndrome identity in clinical practice.

There is some evidence from the main body of research in general psychiatry that persistent depressions over a period of time lead to significant impairment in psychosocial functioning (Geerlings *et al.*, 2002; Petersen *et al.*, 2004). These aggravate physical illnesses (Kennedy & Paykel, 2004a, 2004b) and result in impaired cognitive function (Larsen *et al.*, 2004); they are an independent risk factor in ischemic heart disease and heart failure (Bounhoure, 2006) and in several cardiovascular illnesses (Frasure-Smith, 2008; Hopkins & Brett, 2005); and they influence lifespan by increasing mortality (Bertolote *et al.*, 2003; Plante, 2005). Similarly, they lead to an increase in suicide (Gold *et al.*, 2005; Kiloh *et al.*, 1988). Kendler and colleagues (2005) have demonstrated that there is a difference between S and L carriers regarding sensitivity to stressors. SS individuals have increased sensitivity to mild stresses and experience depression. Thus, they appear to have a demonstrable biological disadvantage (Scadding, 1967). Finally, there are the economic implications as well. Difficult-to-treat depression imposes more than six times the cost of that required to treat a routine patient (Crown *et al.*, 2002; Greenberger *et al.*, 2004; Malhotra *et al.*, 2005; Riso *et al.*, 2002).

To conclude, it is apparent that the TRD field has failed to progress beyond classifications and treatment strategies. This is in spite of the fact that there is increased morbidity and mortality among TRD patients. There is consensus that there exists a definite cohort of patients who do not have personality disorder or another such comorbidity, and yet who experience severe depression and require ongoing ECT or high doses and combinations of antidepressants and other therapies, and continue to not respond to a significant extent. So far there has been no attempt at defining the phenotypic characteristics of these patients by combining or extrapolating the research findings of clinical and neurobiological studies from similar cohorts. To the best of our knowledge, this is the first paper that attempts to do so by examining a large body of data of our own, taken from cohorts with similar psychopathologies.

Towards a new terminology: malignant, pernicious or virulent depression

Morbid and persistent sadness of mood that has deepened to long-standing, recurring depression will be reflected in physical signs including psychomotor retardation and slow mentation, movement and speech. This phenomenon is now well documented in difficult-to-treat melancholic depression (a cohort similar to severe TRD) (Parker, 1995, 2009). Insomnia is another core symptom in recurring and residual depressions (a cohort similar to severe TRD) (Mendlewicz, 2009).

TRD is also associated with nonsuppression by prednisolone (Juruena *et al.*, 2009). The enhanced mineralocorticoid receptor sensitivity normally compensating for glucorticoid resistance is not functional. Consequently, patients with severe depression and TRD demonstrate HPA-axis activity at a high level, with high cortisol levels and impaired negative-feedback response to combined glucocorticoid- and mineralocorticoid-receptor activation by prednisolone.

Hassler and colleagues (2004), in their overview of putative psychopathological and biological endophenotypes, have shown their relevance to the phenotypic definition of major depression. Pharmacogenetic studies provide further impetus to the concept that genetic variants with a high prevalence in the general population probably act to 'promote an organism's resistance to environmental pathogens' (Uhr, 2008). In a similar sense, patients with treatment resistance might resemble a distinct clinical phenotype corresponding to an underlying specific genetic profile. Therefore, the group of patients with narrowly defined malignant, pernicious or virulent depression according to the Maudsley criteria for treatment resistance and to our own definition could serve as a perfect homogeneous population to help in identifying underlying endophenotypes associated with nonresponse and thus further our understanding of therapeutic efficacy in individuals. Since depression in this definition is associated with a pro-inflammatory response, as evidenced by an elevation in C-reactive protein and cytokines such as interleukin-6 and tumour necrosis factor-α, it may soon be possible to include developments such as studies in cytokines (Dinan, 2008). In the long term, the development of a diagnostic system that includes biological and psychopathological endophenotypes is highly desirable, as this would advance research in genetic studies by defining homogenous syndromes in TRD patients.

Another important issue is that of appropriate nomenclature. At present there is considerable discontent regarding the DSM classification and nomenclature system, especially in the context of depressive illnesses. Parker has pointed out that the gravitas added by the prefix 'major' to the term 'depression' distorts the clinical reality and 'subsumes depressive subtypes by its hegemony' (Parker, 2005). Psychiatric diagnosis is considered the weak component of modern research (Angst, 2007; Gupta, 2009) and must find a true phenotype. In a similar vein, Keller *et al.* (2007) have sought to revamp the current diagnostic system, though in the context of psychotic major depression, reflecting dissatisfaction with the current system. Shorter (2007) emphasises several different subtypes of depressive illness and has proposed that the term 'major depression' be replaced by 'melancholic' and 'nonmelancholic' mood disorders.

It would thus appear the time is also ripe to consider a modification of the current nosology of TRD. 'Treatment-resistant' is not a medical term and remains merely an adjective with a subjective flavour to its use in a medical context. The term fails to convey any definite syndrome with an expected clinical picture and outcome. It has come to be associated with a lack of progress in defining putative biological and psychopathological endophenotypes of treatment resistance.

'To name is to know, and a disease known is half cured' runs the proverb. Furthermore, 'the beginning of wisdom is calling things by their right name' (Leahy, 2004). We propose there is wisdom in taking the prefix 'malignant', 'pernicious' or 'virulent' from medicine and calling TRD instead 'malignant depression' or 'pernicious depression' or 'virulent depression'. This would be in step with other medical conditions such as malignant hypertension, pernicious anaemia and virulent infection. In all circumstances, as clinical terms these denote the unremitting or aggressive nature of the underlying illness, its serious clinical ramifications and its relatively poor prognostic outcome. Similarly, virulent, pernicious or malignant depression is associated with increased physical morbidity and increased mortality due to suicide. The very name 'malignant' or 'pernicious' or 'virulent' as a prefix to an illness category generates a concern that requires immediate medical attention, warranting a complete physical examination and clinical investigation. Currently there is nothing to suggest that such concerns are a routine priority for patients with TRD.

We also make the suggestion that the term 'malignant', 'pernicious' or 'virulent' depression may be used for patients who are clearly in the realm of severe TRD, with a cutoff score of 11 or more on the MSM. Such a change in the nomenclature also fits well with Shorter's (2007) suggestion. Treatment-resistant nonpsychotic major depression could be named malignant, pernicious or virulent nonpsychotic depression and treatment-resistant psychotic major depression could be called malignant, pernicious or virulent psychotic depression.

From our data, it is now possible to provide an initial working definition of malignant, pernicious or virulent depression. We found sadness of mood accompanied by hopelessness culminating in suicidal preoccupation/behaviour, insomnia and psychic anxiety the most consistent symptoms and signs among our 18 nonmelancholic but severely treatment-resistant patients. These then form the basis of our proposed definition of malignant depression as a persistent and/or frequently recurring depression despite therapeutic interventions, characterized by profound sadness of mood, hopelessness and suicidal behaviour, insomnia and psychic anxiety clinically reflected in impaired concentration. There is support from several other studies in which these symptoms were also found to be of relevance in serious long-standing depressions; for example, hopelessness in Beck (1990) and Engstrom (1997) and insomnia in Mendlewicz (2009). Similarly, anxiety symptoms form an integral part of serious depression (Fava, 2008; Nemeroff, 2002) and are present in TRD patients (Sourey *et al.*, 2007). Interestingly, six patients who had melancholic TRD (or 'malignant melancholia') differed from the other 18 patients in that they rated significantly high on guilt and self-blame rather than hopelessness. We do not wish these findings in the context of our paper to be confused with the presence of 'psychomotor symptoms' as the cardinal feature in the concept of melancholia

(Parker, 2009). Our suggestion has the advantage that it incorporates both the clinical symptoms and the signs of depression, and that it has the capacity to accommodate new psychobiological advances.

We recognize that overall the number of patients included in developing this definition is small. Malignant, pernicious or virulent depression, as we have described it in this chapter, has the potential to bring together subjective clinical symptoms as well as objective clinical signs, including path physiological research, in similar cohorts of patients. It immediately conveys to us a naturally occurring illness with hardcore symptoms of depression, including increased morbidity and mortality, that arouses concern. Furthermore, the term 'malignant', 'pernicious' or 'virulent' depression has the advantage of not being used as a domain diagnosis, which would include all lifelong miserable people in it. Patients with malignant, pernicious or virulent depression would have a unique clinical profile without overlap of symptoms with other disorders. This is quite unlike the current situation in DSM-IV, where various diagnoses are not mutually exclusive.

Kendler (2009) reminds us that psychiatry is both a science and a practical medical discipline. We must thus allow for the impact of both empirical and pragmatic factors in our nosology. Kendler further continues, 'this is the best way in which psychiatry can follow biology in maturing historically from top down essentialist views of our categories to bottom up empirically defined entities that reflect with increasing accuracy the world as we best understand it'. With therapeutic advances in DBS (Bewermick et al., 2009) and ketamine therapy (Aan Het Rot et al., 2009) in TRD patients, a medical terminology could lead to such a maturation of psychiatry and provide an advantage in dealing with ethical and funding considerations. We invite our colleagues to make similar suggestions so that an appropriate terminology for TRD and its definition can be developed. Our suggestion conforms to McHugh's first cluster of mental disorders, with brain diseases that directly disrupt the neural underpinnings of psychological faculties such as cognition, emotion and perception. Hopefully this step will also be a catalyst in advancing the field towards an aetiopathic understanding.

References

Aan Het Rot, M., Collins, K. A., Murrough, J. W. *et al.* (2010) Safety and efficacy of repeated-dose intravenous ketamine for treatment resistant depression. *Biol. Psychiatry*, **67**(2), 139–145.

Angst, J. (2007) Psychiatric diagnosis: the weak component of modern research. *PMCID*, **6**, 94–95.

Beck, A. T., Brown, G., Berchick, R. J. *et al.* (1990) Relationship between hopelessness and ultimate suicide: a replication with psychiatric outpatients. *Am. J. Psychiatry*, **147**, 190–5.

Berlim, M. T. & Turecki, G. (2007) What is the meaning of treatment resistant/refractory major depression (TRD)? A systematic review of current randomized trials. *Eur. Neuropsychopharmacol.* Epub ahead of print. Available at http://www.ncbi.nlm.nih.gov/pubmed/17521891, last accessed November 9, 2012.

Bertolote, J. M., Fleichmann, A., Leo Diego, D. E. & Wassermann, D. (2003) Suicide and mental disorders: do we know enough? *Brit. J. Psychiatry*, **83**, 383–383.

Bewermick, B. H., Hurleman, R., Mausch, A. *et al.* (2010) Nucleus acumbens deep brain stimulation decreases ratings of depression and anxiety in treatment resistant depression. *Biol. Psychiatry*, **67**(2), 110–116.

Brodaty, H., Luscombe, G., Peisah, C. *et al.* (2001) A 25 years longitudinal, comparison study of depression. *Psy. Med.*, **8**, 1347–1359.

Bounhoure, J. P., Galinier, M., Curnier, D. *et al.* (2006) [Influence of depression on the prognosis of cardiovascular diseases.] *Bull. Acad. Nat. Med.*, **190**(8), 1731–1732.

Burrows, G. D., Norman, T. R. & Judd, F. K. (1994) Definition and differential diagnosis of Treatment Resistant Depression. *Int. Clin. Psychopharmacol.*, **9**(2), 5–10.

Crown, W. H., Finkelstein, S. & Berndt, E. R. (2002) The impact of treatment-resistant depression on health care utilization and costs. *J. Clin. Psychiatry*, **63**(11), 963–971.

Dinan, T. G. (2008) Inflammatory markers in depression. *Curr. Opin. Psychiatry*, **22**, 32–36.

Engstrom, G., Alling, C., Gustavson, P. *et al.* (1997) Clinical characteristics and biological parameters in temperamental cluster of suicide attempters. *J. Affect. Disord.*, **44**, 5–55.

Fava, M. (2003) Diagnosis and definition of treatment-resistant depression. *Biol. Psychiatry*, **53**, 649–659.

Fava, M., Rush, J., Alpert, J. E. *et al.* (2008) Difference in treatment outcome in out patients with anxious versus non anxious patients: a STAR*D report. *Am. J. Psychiatry*, **165**, 342–351.

Fekadu, A., Wooderson, S. C., Donaldson, C. *et al.* (2009) A multidimensional tool to quantify treatment resistance in depression: the Maudsley Staging Method. *J. Clin. Psychiatry*, **70**(2), 177–184.

Fekadu, A., Wooderson, S. C., Kalypso, M. & Cleare, A. J. (2009) The Maudsley Staging Method for treatment-resistant depression: prediction of longer-term outcome and persistence of symptoms. *J. Clin. Psychiatry*, **70**(7), 952–957.

Fleck, M. P. De A., Gregory, S., Herrman, H. *et al.* (2005) Major Depression and its co-relates in primary care setting in six countries. *Brit. J. Psychiatry*, **186**, 41–47.

Fleck, M. P. & Howarth, E. (2005) Pharmacological management of difficult to treat depression in clinical practice. *Psych. Serv.*, **56**(8), 1005–1011.

Frasure-Smith, N. & Lesperance, F. (2008) Depression and anxiety as predictors of 2-year cardiac events in patients with stable coronary artery disease. *Arch. Gen. Psychiatry*, **65**(1), 62–71.

Geerlings, S. W., Beekman, A. T., Deeg, D. J. *et al.* (2002) Duration and severity of depression predict mortality in older adults in the community. *Psy. Med.*, **32**(4), 609–618.

Gold, P. W., Wong, M. L. & Goldstein, D. S. (2005) Cardiac implications of increased arterial entry and reversible 24-h central and peripheral norepinephrine levels in melancholia. *Proc. Natl. Acad. Sci. USA*, **102**(23), 8303–8308.

Greenberger, G. P., Corey-liste, P. K., Birnbaum, H. *et al.* (2004) Economic implications of treatment-resistant depression among employees. *Pharmacoeconomics*, **22**(6), 363–373.

Gupta, R. K. (2009) Major depression: an illness with objective physical signs. *World J. Biol. Psychiatry*, **10**, 196–201.

Hopkins, R. O. & Brett, S. (2005) Chronic neurocognitive effects of critical illness. *Curr. Opin. Crit. Care*, **11**(4), 369–375.

Judd, L. L., Akiskal, H. S., Maser, J. D. *et al.* (1998) A prospective 12-year study of subsyndromal and syndromal depressive symptoms in unipolar major depressive disorders. *Arch. Gen. Psychiatry*, **55**(8), 694–700.

Jurena, M. F., Pariante C. M, Papadopoulos A. S. *et al.* (2009) Prednisolone suppression test in depression: prospective study of the role of HPA axis dysfunction in treatment resistance. *Brit. J. Psychiatry*, **194**, 342–349.

Hasler, G., Drevets W. C., Manji, H. K. & Charney, D. S. (2004) Discovering endophenotypes for major depression. *Neuropsychopharmacol.*, **29**, 1765–1781.

Keller, J., Schatzberg, A. F. & Maj, M. (2007) Current issues in the classification of psychotic major depression. *Schiz. Bull.*, **33**(4), 877–885.

Keller, M. B. (1985) Chronic and recurrent affective disorders: incidence, course, and influencing factors, in *Chronic Treatments in Neuropsychiatry* (ed. D. Kamli & G. Racagni), Raven Press, New York, NY, USA, pp. 68–73.

Keller, M. B., Klerman, G. L., Lavori, P. W. *et al.* (1984) Long term outcome of episodes of major depression. Clinical and public health significance. *JAMA*, **252**, 788–792.

Kendell, R. E. (1975) The concept of disease and its implications for psychiatry. *Brit. J. Psychiatry*, **127**, 305–315.

Kendler, K. S., Kuhn, J. W., Vittum, J. *et al.* (2005) The interaction of stressful life events and a serotonin transporter polymorphism in the prediction of major depression: a replication. *Arch. Gen. Psychiatry*, **62**(5), 529–535.

Kendler, K. S. (2009) An historical frame work for psychiatric nosology. *Psy. Med.*, **39**, 1935–1941.

Kennedy, Y. N. & Paykel, E. S. (2004a) Treatment and response in refractory depression/results from a specialist affective disorder service. *J. Affect. Disord.*, **81**(1), 49–53.

Kennedy, Y. N. & Paykel, E. S. (2004b) Residual symptoms at remission from depression: impact on long-term outcome. *J. Affect. Disord.*, **80**, 135–144.

Kennedy, Y. N., Abbott, R. & Paykel, E. S. (2004) Longitudinal syndromal and sub-syndromal symptoms after severe depression: 10-year follow-up study. *Brit. J. Psychiatry*, **184**, 330–336.

Kielholz, P. (1986) Treatment for therapy resistant depression. *Psychopathology*, **19**(Suppl. 2), 194–200.

Kiloh, L. G., Andrews, G. & Neilson, M. (1988) The long term outcome of depressive illness. *Brit. J. Psychiatry*, **153**, 752–757.

Klein, N., Sacher, J., Wallner, H. *et al.* (2004) Therapy of treatment resistant depression: focus on the management of TRD with atypical antipsychotics. *CNS Spectrum*, **11**, 823–832.

Kupfer, D. J. & Charney, D. S. (2003) Difficult-to-treat depression. *Biol. Psychiatry*, **53**, 633–634.

Laing, R. D. (1967) *The Politics of Experience*, Penguin Books.

Larson, S. L., Clark, M. R. & Eaton, W. W. (2004) Depressive disorder as a long-term antecedent risk factor for incident back pain: a 13-year follow-up study from Baltimore Epidemiological Catchment Area Sample. *Psy. Med.*, **34**, 211–219.

Leahy, C. W. (2004) *The Birdwatcher's Companion to North American Birdlife*, Princeton University Press, Princeton, NJ, USA.

Licht-Strunk, E., Van Marwijk, H. W., Twisk, J. W. *et al.* (2009) Outcome of depression in later life in primary care: longitudinal cohort study with three years' follow-up. *BMJ*, **338**, 3079.

Malhi, G. S., Parker, G. B., Crawford, J. G. *et al.* (2005) Treatment-resistant depression: resistant to definition? *Acta Psychiatr. Scand.*, **112**(4), 302–309.

Malhotra, A. K., Murphy, G. M. & Kennedy, J. L. (2004) Pharma-cogenetics of psychotopic drugs and response. *Am. J. Psychiatry*, **161**(5), 780–791.

Mendlewicz, J. (2009) Sleep disturbances: core symptoms of major depressive disorder rather than associated or comorbid disorders. *World J. Biol. Psychiatry*, **10**, 1–7.

McHugh, P. R. (2005) Striving for coherence, psychiatry's efforts over classification. *JAMA*, **293**(20), 2526–2528.

Mitchell, A. J., Vaze, A. & Rao, S. (2009) Clinical diagnosis of depression in primary care: a meta-analysis. *Lancet*, **374**(9690), 609–619.

Möller, H.-J. (2009) Antidepressants: controversies about the efficacy in depression, their effect on suicidality and their place in complex psychiatric treatment approach. *World J. Biol. Psychiatry*, **10**(3), 180–195.

Nemeroff, C. B. (2002) Comorbidity of mood and anxiety disorders: the rule, not the exception? *Am. J. Psychiatry*, **159**, 3–4.

Parker, G. (1995) Subtyping depression II. Clinical distinction of psychotic depression and non psychotic melancholia. *Psy. Med.*, **25**, 825–835.

Parker, G. (2005) Beyond major depression. *Psy. Med.*, **35**, 467–474.

Parker, G. (2008) How should mood disorders be modelled? *Aus. NZ J. Psychiatry*, **42**(10), 841–850.

Parker, G. B., Malhi, G. S., Crawford, J. G. & Thase, M. E. (2005) Identifying 'paradigm failures' contributing to treatment-resistant depression. *J. Affect. Disord.*, **87**, 185–191.

Parker, G., Fletcher, K., Hyett, M. *et al.* (2009) Measuring melancholia: the utility of a prototypic symptom approach. *Psy. Med.*, **39**, 989–998.

Petersen, T., Papakostas, G. I., Mahal, Y. *et al.* (2004) Psychosocial functioning in patients with treatment resistant depression. *Eur. Psychiatry*, **19**(4), 196–201.

Petersen, T., Papakostas, G. I., Posternak, M. A. *et al.* (2005) Empirical testing of two models for staging antidepressant treatment resistance. *J. Clin. Psychopharmacol.*, **25**(4), 336–341.

Phillips, K. & Nierenberg, G. A. A. (1994) The assessment and treatment of refractory depression. *J. Clin. Psychiatry*, **55**(Suppl. 2), 20–26.

Plante, G. E. (2005) Depression and cardiovascular disease: a reciprocal relationship. *Metabolism*, **54**(5 Suppl. 1), 45–48.

Riso, L. P., Miyatake, R. K. & Thase, M. E. (2002) The search for determinants of chronic depression: a review of six factors. *J. Affect. Disord.*, **70**(2), 103–115.

Robins, E. & Guze, S. D. (1972) Classification of affective disorders: the primary-secondary, the endogenous-reactive and the neurotic-psychotic, in *Recent Advances of Psychobiology of Depressive Illnesses* (ed. T. A. Williams, M. M. Katz & J. A. Shields), Printing Office, Washington, DC, USA.

Scadding, J. G. (1967) Diagnosis: the clinician and the computer. *Lancet*, **ii**, 1085–1093.

Scott, J. (1988) Chronic depression. *Brit. J. Psychiatry*, **153**, 287–297.

Shorter, E. (2007) The doctorine of two depressions in historical perspective. *Acta Psychiatr. Scand.*, **115**, 5–13.

Sourey, D., Amsterdam, J., de Montigny, C. *et al.* (1999) Treatment resistant depression: methodological overview and operational criteria. *Eur. Neuropsychopharmacol.*, **9**, 83–91.

Souery, D., Papakostas, G. I. & Trivedi, M. H. (2006) Treatment-resistant depression. *J. Clin. Psychiatry*, **67**(6), 16–22.

Sourey, D., Oswald, P., Massat, I. *et al.* (2007) Group for the Study of Resistant Depression (2007) Clinical factors associated with treatment resistance in major depressive disorder: results from a European multicenter study. *J. Clin. Psychiatry*, **68**(7), 1062–1070.

Taylor, K. (1971) A Logical analysis of the medico-psychological concept of disease. *Psy. Med.*, **1**, 356–364.

Thase, M. E. & Rush, A. J. (1995) Treatment resistant depression. In *Psychopharmacology: The Fourth Generation of Progress* (ed. F. E. Bloom & D. J. Kupfer), Raven Press, New York, NY, USA.

Thase, M. E. & Rush, A. J. (1997) When at first you don't succeed: sequential strategies for antidepressant nonresponders. *J. Clin. Psychiatry*, **58**(13), 23–29.

Thomson, F. & Craighead, M. (2008) Innovative approaches for the treatment of depression: targeting the HPA axis. *Neurochem. Res.*, **33**, 691–707.

Robinson, O. J. & Sahakian, B. J. (2008) Recurrence in major depressive disorder: a neurocognitive perspective. *Psy. Med.*, **38**, 315–318.

Uhr, M., Tontsch, A., Namendorf, C. *et al.* (2008) Polymorphisms in the drug transporter gene ABCB1gene predict antidepressant treatment response in depression. *Neuron*, **57**, 203–209.

Zimmerman, M., Chelminski, I., McGlinchey, J. B. & Young, D. (2006) Diagnosing major depressive disorder X; can the utility of the DSM-IV symptom criteria be improved. *J. Nerv. Ment. Dis.*, **194**(12), 893–897.

CHAPTER 3

Genetics of Treatment-resistant Depression

Chiara Fabbri, Stefano Porcelli
and Alessandro Serretti
*Department of Biomedical and NeuroMotor Sciences,
University of Bologna, Bologna, Italy*

Summary

Gene variants influence the clinical outcomes of antidepressant treatments, explaining 50% of the variance. In particular, treatment-resistant depression (TRD) is a cause of considerable societal burden and would greatly benefit from the identification of genetic predictors. The most promising genes for association with TRD are SLC6A4, 5-HTR1A, COMT, BDNF and CREB1, but further work is needed in order to translate findings into clinical recommendations. Indeed, the complex nature of major depression and antidepressant response make the picture complex to dissect. Nonetheless, hopefully in a few years, genetic prediction of TRD could become a widespread clinical reality.

Introduction

Available evidence consistently demonstrates that major depressive disorder (MDD) has a strong genetic background, an idea

Treatment-resistant Depression, First Edition. Edited by Siegfried Kasper
and Stuart Montgomery.

which finds its roots in ancient times. Indeed, Hippocrates was the first to describe the constitutional-type theory and to observe the recurrence of mental disease in the same families. These observations led to the idea of 'atavism', the reappearance in an individual of a trait after several generations of absence. Despite the ancient origin of this theory, it was only at the beginning of the 20th century that the first twin studies were performed; today, thanks to studies in monozygotic and dizygotic twins, the heredit-ability of MDD is considered to be at least 37% (Sullivan *et al.*, 2000). In the 1990s it became clear that the disease showed not only a familiar clustering but also a familiar aggregation of response to treatment. Mechanisms linked to the pathophysiology of mood disorders are hypothesized to be similar to those involved in drug response within the same familiar cluster (Serretti *et al.*, 1998). Subsequent studies unearthed increasing evidence of the contribution of genetic factors to antidepressant response, which is estimated at 50% or more (Maier & Zobel, 2008).

These promising findings suggested that the genes underly-ing the pathophysiology of depression and antidepressant response could be detected, leading to the birth of pharmacoge-netics, the research field dealing with the detection of genetic predictors of treatment response and drug-related adverse events, with the aim of improving disease outcome. It is well known that approximately 99.5% of the genome DNA sequence is identical among humans, so the remaining 0.5% is account-able for individual differences, including both susceptibility to diseases and drug response. This difference consists of di-, tri- and tetra- nucleotide repeats (satellite sequences), large vari-ants >1 kbp due to deletions, insertions or duplications (copy number variants, CNVs) and nucleotide substitutions. There are 7 million substitutions in each individual human genome, and over 80% of them take the form of single-nucleotide polymor-phisms (SNPs), so SNPs account for over 80% of the variability between humans, including disease predisposition (Roberts *et al.*, 2010). Today the HapMap project allows easy research into SNPs; it has currently mapped the location of over 3 million (http://hapmap.ncbi.nlm.nih.gov/).

The first pharmacogenetic studies were based on the candidate gene approach; that is, the analysis of genetic variants selected *a priori* on the basis of preclinical data. Genes selected through this method are those coding for key molecular components of the serotoninergic, noradrenergic and dopaminergic systems, which functional abnormalities are thought to be the basis of MDD pathophysiology. Their restoration may be a consequence of antidepressant treatment. According to the monoaminergic theory, MDD is caused by a decreased monoaminergic function in the brain (although this is without a doubt an oversimplification) (Porcelli *et al.*, 2011a). Thus, the serotonin transporter gene (SLC6A4), serotonin 1A receptor (5-HT1A), serotonin 2A receptor (5-HT2A), tryptophan hydroxylase 1 and 2 (TPH1, TPH2), catechol-O-methyltransferase (COMT), monoamine oxidase A (MAOA) and norepinephrine transporter (SLC6A2) were considered among the best *a priori* candidate genes. Nonetheless, given the inconsistency of findings obtained by the candidate gene approach, it became clear that the genetic component of antidepressant response was likely linked to a number of genes, each with a small effect size, rather than to one or a few major loci. On the other hand, the high rates of incomplete treatment response or true treatment-resistant depression (TRD) and the high early discontinuation rates due to side effects made it necessary to find sensitive and specific predictors of clinical outcomes. With this aim, more recent pharmacogenetic studies have tried to increase the coverage of the genetic variability to the whole genome, through the genome-wide association approach (genome-wide association studies or GWASs). GWASs, through the use of microarray technology, allow wide coverage of the genetic variability associated with a phenotype. They overcome the need for any *a priori* hypothesis – a very useful tool in this field, since antidepressant mechanisms of action are not fully understood. Furthermore, biological plausibility is not an initial requirement for a convincing statistical association, as there are many examples in human genetics of previously unsuspected candidate genes nonetheless showing highly compelling associations (Psychiatric GWAS Consortium

Steering Committee, 2009). GWASs have already produced promising results in the study of other complex diseases, such as coronary artery disease, type 1 and 2 diabetes and rheumatoid arthritis (Wellcome Trust Case Control Consortium, 2007), showing them to be a powerful method for the detection of genes involved in common human diseases.

With regard to antidepressant response, unfortunately inconsistent results have been found, probably due to some unsolved methodological and technical issues. Among these are some technical limitations which do not allow rare genetic variants to be detected, inadequate sample sizes (our current knowledge suggests that future GWASs will need samples of tens of thousands, rather than the thousands traditionally used) and the still inaccurate phenotype definition. Moreover, the effect of a number of stratification factors might be a further source of bias (Serretti *et al.*, 2008). Strategies to solve these issues are already emerging. Indeed, nowadays pharmacogenetic studies collect more and more detailed clinical data for use in the analysis together with genetic information, and the use of large replication samples is now possible thanks to the growth of controlled-access data repositories via the NIMH Human Genetics Initiative (http://nimhgenetics.org). Finally, technical improvements in and a reduction in the costs of genotyping are also expected.

We cannot exclude the possibility that GWASs may not be the best tool by which to detect the loci associated with antidepressant response, since the multiple loci with small effect sizes likely involved in antidepressant effect may not be detectable in realistic sample sizes with alpha error at a genome-wide level of significance (10^{-7}–10^{-8}), and heterogeneity within and between samples reduces the chance of reaching this threshold and replicating findings. Hence, GWASs may be more useful as a complement to other approaches (e.g. sequencing of candidate genes, pathway analysis).

Given the results of candidate gene studies and GWASs, different neuronal systems probably act behind the pathophysiology of MDD and antidepressant effect. The aim of the present chapter is to link these findings with the main current hypothesis of MDD pathophysiology in order to underline the basic mechanisms of antidepressant response/resistance. Each finding is likely one piece of a very complex picture. Indeed, MDD may be the result of several different pathological mechanisms, which result in a common phenotype, as well as a complex interaction among several systems, which may sustain different depressive symptoms. In the following sections we will focus on the main systems supposed to be involved in MDD, with the aim of closing the gap between the main hypothesis of MDD pathogenesis and our current pharmacogenetic knowledge.

Genetic polymorphisms and antidepressant efficacy

Antidepressant pharmacodynamics

Monoaminergic system

The monoaminergic theory of MDD led the research into the disease over the last few decades. It has its roots in the 1950s in the clever clinical observation that some compounds, such as iproniazid and imipramine, share the property of influencing the balance of monoamines in the central nervous system (CNS) and show unexpected antidepressant effects. On the other hand, reserpine, an old antihypertensive agent that depletes monoamine stores, is able to produce depressive symptoms. Hence, according to the monoaminergic theory, MDD develops as a result of an insufficiency of noradrenergic, dopaminergic or serotonergic neurotransmission. On the basis of this theory, the majority of the currently available antidepressants were developed, with only some exceptions (e.g. agomelatine).

   Nonetheless, since the introduction of the first drugs that act through enhancement of the monoaminergic system, it has become clear that this theory fails to completely elucidate the pathophysiology of MDD. Indeed, several issues are not explained by the monoaminergic theory: first, despite the rapid enhancement of monoaminergic transmission, the antidepressant effect appears only after some weeks of treatment; second, monoamine depletion does not decrease mood in healthy subjects, although it does slightly decrease mood in healthy subjects with a family history of depression (Porcelli *et al.*, 2011a); third, a subgroup of depressed patients does not respond to monoaminergic antidepressants. Given these issues, it has been hypothesized that the homeostasis of the monoaminergic system may play a role in the delayed onset of the antidepressant response; that is, the system may respond to external enhancement with an early downregulation of transmission, while only the later synaptic plasticity leads to an increase in transmission. This hypothesis is supported by the detection of presynaptic autoreceptors with inhibitory function – 5-HTR1A – whose antagonism has been reported to shorten the antidepressant effect. However, this may explain the lag before the delayed clinical effect of monoaminergic antidepressants, but it does not address other concerns about the monoaminergic theory, such as the lack of response in a subgroup of patients. It has been hypothesized that genetics may at least partially account for these unsolved issues. Thus, a number of studies have investigated the genetic variants which may explain why the enhancement of the monoaminergic system is not enough for all patients suffering from MDD.

The first genes to be investigated pertain to the serotonin system, due to the great evidence for its involvement in the pathophysiology of MDD. Among them, the most investigated is the serotonin transporter gene (SLC6A4). Given the hypothesis that a reduced serotoninergic transmission may cause MDD, the blocking of the serotonin transporter (SERT, the main target of antidepressant drugs and the principal site of action of selective serotonin reuptake inhibitors (SSRIs)) by antidepressant drugs should lead to recovery, thanks to an increase in serotonin availability at the synaptic level. Indeed, SERT regulates brain serotonin neurotransmission by transporting the neurotransmitter serotonin from the synaptic cleft to presynaptic neurons. The most investigated variant within the SLC6A4 gene is without a doubt the 44 bp insertion/deletion polymorphism (5-HTTLPR) at the promoter of the gene, which has been reported to affect gene expression. The polymorphism is a sequence of repeated elements: the 16-repeat sequence is called the long allele (L) and shows a twice-basal SERT expression compared to the 11-repeat sequence (short allele or S). Most pharmacogenetic studies demonstrate a lower antidepressant response in S carriers, particularly for SSRIs (Porcelli *et al.*, 2011b). In the light of the monoaminergic theory of MDD, these findings suggest that in L carriers the blocking of the SERT by antidepressant drugs may be enough to produce a clinical effect, while in S carriers it may be insufficient.

What is the reason behind this discrepancy? Preclinical and clinical data may help to solve this matter: several studies have reported that SERT knockout (KO) mice show a behavioural phenotype reminiscent of some symptoms of MDD, such as inhibited exploratory locomotion, increased anxiety, reduced aggressive behaviour and reduced home-cage activity. Moreover, in humans, imaging studies show that S carriers have higher levels of amygdala activity and reduced functional coupling of the amygdala–anterior cingulate cortex (ACC) circuit (Scharinger *et al.*, 2011), phenotypes associated with anxiety and MDD. These findings clearly suggest that the lack of SERT produces a behavioural phenotype similar to MDD; thus a reduction of SERT activity may produce endophenotypes related to a higher risk of MDD. What do these data mean in the light of the monoaminergic theory? It has been hypothesized that a reduction of basal SERT activity may lead to an inadequate synaptic serotonin reuptake and therefore to inadequate presynaptic serotonin storage, since it becomes largely dependent on serotonin production. This condition may consequently lead to a lower presynaptic ability to release serotonin after repeated stimulations. In other words, S carriers may display a lower ability to respond to repeated releasing inputs, and the consequent reduction of serotoninergic transmission may be linked to an increased risk of MDD. Although this hypothesis may account for the higher risk of MDD shown by S carriers, it does not clarify why they show a worse response to SSRIs. A possible explanation is that in L carriers the defect which leads to MDD is an inadequate persistence of serotonin at the synaptic level, at least partially due to an excessive SERT function. The blocking of SERT in these subjects may be enough to produce the antidepressant effect, since it causes an increased persistence of serotonin into the synaptic cleft and, consequently, an increased stimulation of postsynaptic receptors. On the other hand, in S carriers the defect that leads to MDD may be a reduced presynaptic storage of serotonin, so serotonin reuptake blockage might cause a further reduction of the presynaptic storage and, consequently, a further reduction of the synaptic ability to respond to repeated stimuli. Furthermore, the effect of SSRIs on the synaptic persistence of serotonin may be less important in S carriers because of the high basal synaptic serotonin persistence. From this point of view, data concerning 5-HTR1A may provide further elucidation of these hypotheses.

The 5-HT1A receptor is abundant in corticolimbic regions and can be expressed both pre- and postsynaptically. At the level of the serotonin cell bodies in the midbrain dorsal raphe nucleus, it acts as an autoreceptor, inhibiting the firing of serotonin neurons and reducing the release of serotonin (5-HT) in the prefrontal cortex. In other words, 5HT1A autoreceptors help to maintain the homeostasis of serotoninergic transmission, activating a feedback control on presynaptic serotonin release. How does this receptor interact with different levels of SERT activity? We could hypothesize that the effect of 5-HT1A autoreceptors is relevant in L carriers, particularly at the beginning of antidepressant treatment. Indeed, the increase of serotonin persistence at the synaptic level caused by SSRIs stimulates the 5-HT1A autoreceptor and, therefore, the inhibition of the firing of serotonin neurons. After some weeks of treatment, this negative feedback gradually disappears and the antidepressant effect becomes clinically detectable. At the beginning of treatment, the mechanisms involved in this dynamic adaptation are probably 5-HTR1A internalization and degradation, while subsequently DNA transcription and epigenetic changes at the 5-HTR1A locus occur. On the other hand, the effects of the 5-HTR1A stimulation may last for a longer time in S carriers, showing a slower adaptation, since SSRI intake does not result in a stronger 5-HT release or a longer 5-HT persistence at the synaptic level. In these subjects (or better, in a greater part of them) serotonergic antidepressants probably lead only to a small global increase of the serotonin transmission, enough to activate the 5-HT1A autoreceptor but not to determinate the dynamic adaptation seen in L carriers (alternatively, this adaptation may require more time in S carriers). Therefore, the effect of 5-HTR1A may be more deleterious in S carriers, and may partially account for the worse antidepressant response. This hypothesis is supported by studies on pindolol, a 5-HTR1A antagonist used as an augmentation to antidepressants, since it seems to speed up their clinical effect. Interestingly, some studies on TRD patients have reported that S carriers show better improvement during pindolol augmentation, supporting the idea that 5-HTR1A adaptation does not occur (or occurs more slowing/less frequently) in S carriers (Porcelli *et al.*, 2011c).

The picture becomes more complex when we consider that the expression of 5-HTR1A is affected by genetic variants. Among these, the most investigated SNP is the rs6295 (1019C/G), which G allele results in an upregulation of the gene. Theoretically, the rs6295 G allele should contrast the enhancement of the serotoninergic transmission with a higher number of presynaptic inhibitory 5-HT1A receptors (Porcelli *et al.*, 2011c). This hypothesis is supported by preclinical data. Indeed, in mice the rise of 5-HT1A autoreceptor levels leads to depressive behaviour (Albert & Francois, 2010), while their reduction prior to antidepressant treatment is enough to convert nonresponders into responders (Richardson-Jones *et al.*, 2010). Several studies have consistently suggested the G allele is a risk factor for TRD, although negative results exist as well (Porcelli *et al.*, 2011c). 5-HT1A receptors are also expressed postsynaptically, with a different – and not completely understood – function. Some interesting suggestions concerning this function come from preclinical studies on 5-HTR1A KO mice. These mice display increased anxiety behaviour and are unresponsive to SSRI treatment. On the other hand, early 5-HTR1A overexpression during development seems to decrease anxiety. Thus, a rise in 5-HT1A autoreceptors seems to lead to MDD and to SSRI resistance, while a reduction in postsynaptic 5-HT1A receptors seems to be implicated in anxiety behaviours. Imaging human studies show consistent reductions in postsynaptic 5-HT1A receptors in subsets of prefrontal and temporal cortical regions in both depressive and anxiety disorders, while 5-HT1A autoreceptor levels were increased in MDD.

In summary, both a lower SERT function (e.g. due to the S allele of 5-HTTLPR) and an overexpression of 5-HT1A autoreceptors (e.g. due to the G allele of rs6295) may lead to poor antidepressant response, but through different mechanisms. The effect of these two deleterious alleles may be even worse when they coexist in the same subject, probably resulting in TRD.

5-HTTLPR and rs6295 are the most investigated polymorphisms within the SLC6A4 and 5-HTR1A genes, but several other variants have also been reported to affect their expression and functionality. Therefore, although the concepts discussed in this section hold true, we must keep in mind that the real picture is even more complex. For example, within the SLC6A4 gene, other relevant variants associated with transporter expression/activity include the rs25531 and a 17 bp VNTR (variable number of tandem repeats) identified within intron 2 (STin2) (Porcelli *et al.*, 2011c). Although these variants have not been well investigated so far, they may account for the partial inconsistency among the different pharmacogenetic studies, at least in part. Thus, further investigations are required to allow us to better understand their effects.

Another relevant player within the serotonin synapses is one of the main postsynaptic serotonin receptors, the 5-HT2A receptor (5HTR2A) – a G-coupled postsynaptic receptor with widespread distribution throughout the cortex and high densities in the frontal cortex. An increasing amount of evidence suggests that 5-HTR2A is also involved in MDD pathophysiology and antidepressant mechanisms of action. In particular, drugs with agonist proprieties to 5-HTR2A show euphoriant effects and various antidepressants affect 5-HT2A receptor binding activity (Porcelli *et al.*, 2011c). Interestingly, the receptor binding profile alone seems to be relevant to MDD pathophysiology and antidepressant effect. Indeed, a growing body of evidence suggests a decreased cortical 5-HT2A receptor binding in MDD patients compared with healthy controls (Dhaenen, 2001). The duration of the illness appears to be related to this feature: in first-episode subjects, no difference has been found compared to healthy controls, while TRD patients show lower 5-HT2A receptor binding in the dorsal regions of the prefrontal cortex and the ACC. Drug-naïve patients not at onset show a similar 5-HTR2A downregulation, suggesting that this state is not caused by a long antidepressant treatment but is likely a depressive trait related to the duration of the illness. On the other hand, successful treatment response with SSRIs and electroconvulsive therapy (ECT) is associated with prefrontal 5-HT2A receptor upregulation. Therefore, reversal of the 5-HTR2A downregulation may be needed in order to achieve the antidepressant effect. The reason why this does not occur in TRD is an open field of research. Some authors suggest that the reduced cortical 5-HT2A receptor binding found in TRD patients might be due to the prefrontal neurodegenerative effects secondary to hypercortisolaemia in long-term depressed states. Nonetheless, it is not clear why this degenerative process cannot be stopped and, eventually, reversed by antidepressant treatment in TRD, as happens in non-TRD patients. Perhaps the answer once more lies in genetics, at least partially. In particular, focusing on rs6311 (-1438G/A) within the 5-HTR2A gene, a SNP which has received great attention in recent years, may help us to better understand this issue. rs6311 is a G-to-A sequence variation at the promoter which results in the loss of a CpG site, a methylation site involved in the epigenetic mechanisms of gene-expression regulation. Moreover, this site is a binding position for transcription factors and the transcriptional activator E47 binds selectively to the A allele at position -1438 (Falkenberg *et al.*, 2011). Therefore, the presence of the A allele does not allow methylation at this site (a mechanism of gene silencing) and promotes binding of the transcriptional activator E47, resulting in a higher gene expression of 5-HTR2A. Taking into account that a 5-HTR2A downregulation may be related to MDD and TRD, the presence of the A allele may be associated with a better antidepressant response and may be protective for TRD. Some authors have shown an association between antidepressant response and rs6311. Further, a recent metaanalysis concluded that rs6311 was associated with SSRI treatment response, but not with other classes of antidepressant (Kato & Serretti, 2010). Nonetheless, so far the allele responsible for the risk of antidepressant resistance has not been elucidated, and further studies are needed in order to confirm the association of the A allele with better antidepressant response. Obviously, there are other genetic variants within the 5-HTR2A gene that might modulate its expression/functionality (e.g. rs7997012), justifying the controversial results concerning rs6311, but further studies are clearly required. In any case, we might hypothesize that every variant which leads to a lower 5-HTR2A expression/functionality should theoretically be associated with worse antidepressant response and TRD.

So far we have focused on serotonin transmission, but another key point in the serotonin system is the biosynthesis of serotonin itself. Indeed, key enzymes involved in the metabolism of monoamines also play a role in the regulation of their balance in the CNS. With regard to serotonin biosynthesis, the limiting step is catalysed by tryptophan hydroxylase (TPH), which is codified by two distinct genes, TPH1 and TPH2. TPH1 is ubiquitous but predominantly expressed in peripheral organs, while TPH2 is more selectively expressed in the brain. TPH2 KO mice show reduced serotonin tone in the CNS, while TPH1 KO mice do not show this alteration (Porcelli *et al.*, 2011c). The initial rationale behind investigating these genes as predictors of antidepressant response derived from the hypothesis that a reduced basal serotonin synthesis might be a risk factor for MDD. In agreement with this, the first pharmacogenetic studies on TPH1 suggested an association between a decreased TPH1 enzyme activity due to the rarer A allele of rs1800532, worse antidepressant response and suicidal behaviour. Unfortunately, further studies failed to replicate these results, showing contradictory findings. Concerning the TPH2 gene, two SNPs (arginine441/proline447 and 1463G/A) have been associated with a reduction in serotonin synthesis, with the latter being found to modulate the fluoxetine response, although only by one preliminary study. Other polymorphisms within the TPH2 gene have been associated with antidepressant response (e.g. rs1386494, rs1487276, rs10897346 and rs1487278), but their effects on the expression/functionality of the enzyme are still under investigation and results are largely controversial. On the other hand, both preclinical and clinical studies suggest an effect of antidepressant treatment on TPH transcription. In particular, an upregulation of TPH following antidepressant treatment has been reported for both TPH1 and TPH2. Furthermore, in humans, higher levels of TPH2 mRNA and protein have been found in the raphe nuclei of MDD patients who committed suicide, suggesting a possible homeostatic response to deficient serotonin levels in the brain of depressed suicides. Intriguingly, some authors found that antidepressant treatment may normalize this basal upregulation of TPH2 expression (Porcelli *et al.*, 2011c). In summary, on one hand a reduced basal TPH activity due to genetic variants may be a risk factor for MDD and worse response to antidepressants; on the other, the increase of TPH expression may be a homeostatic response to a reduced serotonin tone during depressive states. Hence, upregulation of the TPH gene may be required in order to reach the antidepressant effect. In other words, the upregulation found in both suicide victims and depressed patients during antidepressant treatment may be part of the recovery process, regardless of whether it happens spontaneously or following treatment. After recovery, the upregulation may reverse to the basal condition, according to the normalization of the TPH expression found following antidepressant treatment. The genetic variants that are able to interfere with these dynamic adaptations of the TPH expression (e.g. functional SNPs that reduce the enzyme transcription/functionality such as TPH1 rs1800532) may lead to TRD, affecting a key step in the recovery process.

So far we have focused on the serotoninergic system and analysed how genetic variants within the genes coding for the SERT, the presynaptic and postsynaptic receptors and the key enzyme involved in serotonin biosynthesis may lead to TRD. In the CNS, the serotoninergic system is deeply interrelated with the other monoaminergic circuits (Figure 3.1). Therefore, the genetic variants reported so far will likely interact with polymorphisms within key noradrenergic and dopaminergic genes (but probably also with genes harboured by other brain systems), producing the final clinical phenotype. Among these genes, the most relevant with regard to antidepressant pharmacogenetics include MAOA and COMT, which code for enzymes involved in the catabolism of monoamines. Monoamine oxidase (MAO) is a family of enzymes with a key role in the inactivation of neurotransmitters and a direct impact on the regulation of their levels in the brain. In humans, two distinct isoforms are expressed: MAOA, which is the most investigated in psychiatry and mainly breaks serotonin, norepinephrine and epinephrnine; and MAOB, which is mainly investigated with regard to its role in Parkinson's disease and mainly breaks phenethylamine and benzylamine. Both forms break dopamine equally. The first evidence of an influence of MAOA activity on human behaviour derived from the discovery of a syndrome characterized by borderline mental retardation and impulsive aggression, attempted rape and exhibitionism in carriers of a punctual non-sense (i.e. resulting in a truncated protein without its native function) MAOA mutation (Porcelli et al., 2011c). MAOA KO mice display elevated brain concentrations of dopamine, serotonin and noradrenaline and manifest aggressive behaviour. On the other hand, MAOB KO mice do not exhibit aggression and display only high levels of phenylethylamine (Shih et al., 1999).

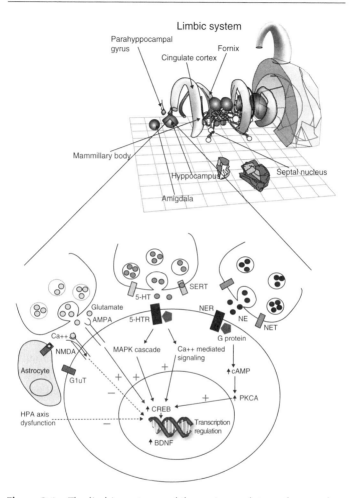

Figure 3.1   The limbic system and the main regulators of neuroplasticity. The focus is on the hippocampus, since neuroplasticity processes have mainly been studied at this level, but other brain areas are also involved (e.g. the prefrontal cortex). SERT, serotonin transporter; NET, norepinephrine transporter; GluT, glutamate transporter; 5-HTR, serotonin receptor; NER, norepinephrine receptor; PKCA, protein kinase C alpha

The role of MAOA in MDD pathophysiology and antidepressant response is largely supported by the clinical effectiveness of MAOA inhibitors (MAOIs), and pharmacogenetics has provided some interesting findings. One particular polymorphism within the MAOA gene has been deeply investigated: a 30 bp VNTR, located 1.2 kb upstream in the MAOA coding sequence, which seems to influence the transcription rate of the gene. Alleles with three and a half or four copies of the repeat sequence are transcribed two to ten times more efficiently than those with three or five copies of the repeat, suggesting an optimal length for the regulatory region (Porcelli *et al.*, 2011c). Nonetheless, the impact on the enzyme activity *in vivo* is not uniformly established. Some suggestions derive from imaging studies: in particular, carriers of long alleles show higher amygdala reactivity in response to aversive stimuli (a trait similar to that found in 5-HTTLPR S carriers) and increase functional coupling of a neural pathway between the ventromedial prefrontal cortex and the amygdala, which is associated with higher levels of harm avoidance, a dimension of the Temperament and Character Inventory (TCI) related to MDD. Overall, long alleles have been associated with both a higher risk of MDD and a poorer antidepressant efficacy (Porcelli *et al.*, 2011c). Thus, an excessive MAO activity may increase the risk of both MDD and worse antidepressant response. Nonetheless, pharmacogenetic findings are not univocal and the specific molecular effect of this mutation is not yet fully understood; nor are the roles of other variants within the gene. Furthermore, the MAOA gene is localized on the X chromosome, so the effect of this polymorphism may be different between the genders, as suggested by some studies. Further investigation is clearly needed in order to better understand the role of this gene and its mutations. Finally, we must remember that the picture is even more complex given the high number of genetic variants within related genes (e.g. dopaminergic and noradrenergic transporter genes), which likely interact with MAOA to produce molecular effects.

Beyond MAO, the catechol-O-methyltransferase (COMT) gene seems to be involved in MDD pathophysiology and antidepressant response, with a key role in monoamine reduction. Two different transcription sites are responsible for the production of the soluble cytoplasmic (S-COMT) and membrane-bound (MB-COMT) COMT isoform. MB-COMT is believed to be the dominant isoform in the brain, whereas S-COMT predominates in the periphery. MB-COMT assumes a greater level of importance in the frontal cortex and in the striatal neurons postsynaptic to the dopaminergic neurons, because it is responsible for more than 60% of dopamine degradation in these sites. Multiple interactions are thought to link the dopaminergic and serotoninergic systems, resulting in reciprocal crosstalking and regulation. Indeed, in animal models of MDD, decreased availability of extracellular dopamine in the nucleus accumbens has been found to be reversible on treatment with serotonergic antidepressants; such a reversal is accompanied by improvements in depressive-like behaviour. Reciprocally, blockade of dopamine D2/D3 receptors acutely reverses the antidepressant effect of SSRIs in MDD animal models, as well as in humans. It has been hypothesized that the effects on the dopaminergic system may represent the final common step of the several mechanisms likely involved in MDD pathophysiology and the final target of any antidepressant treatment (Porcelli *et al.*, 2011a).

In the field of antidepressant pharmacogenetics, one SNP within the COMT gene has received particular attention: Val108/158Met (rs4680). This variant shows a relevant functional effect: the Val/Val genotype catabolizes dopamine at up four times the rate of Met/Met homozygote, resulting in a significant reduction of synaptic dopamine following neurotransmitter release. This polymorphism may not simply affect the synaptic dopamine levels but also impact on serotoninergic activity. Nonetheless, the investigation into its role in antidepressant response has so far failed to find any univocal results (Porcelli *et al.*, 2011c), probably because several stratification factors alter its effects. Indeed, the results are less controversial when we focus on a particular subgroup of MDD, such as TRD. For example, some studies have found an association between the Val allele and better ECT response, suggesting that the development of an antidepressant effect in patients with lower dopamine availability may require other mechanisms beyond an enhancement of monoaminergic transmission. Nonetheless, this hypothesis remains only a speculation until further studies can clarify the effect of this variant, as well as the effects of other variants which have recently emerged (e.g. rs2075507 and rs165599).

Despite the great relevance of the monoaminergic system to MDD pathogenesis, it cannot completely explain either the complex nature of the disease or the mechanisms of action of antidepressants. The monoaminergic theory likely represents one piece of a very complex puzzle, involving other brain systems such as the glutamatergic system and the neurotrophin pathway. From this point of view, the lack of antidepressants with alternative mechanisms of action may account for the incomplete efficacy of current treatments.

Glutamatergic system

Increasing evidence suggests that the glutamatergic system may play a role in MDD pathogenesis and in the mechanisms of the antidepressant response. Glutamate is the main excitatory neurotransmitter in the CNS and its molecular effects are mediated through both ionotropic receptors (NMDA, AMPA and kainate receptors) and receptors linked to intracellular second messenger systems (metabotropic or mGlu). The glutamatergic theory posits that glutamate may shape the risk of MDD influencing neuronal fate (neurotoxicity due to excess influx of Ca^{++} through the NMDA receptor) or the unfolding of new neuronal nets (neuroplasticity). The greatest evidence of imbalance in the glutamatergic signalling has been demonstrated in the hippocampus, where it is likely involved in stress-induced neuronal atrophy and death in the CA3 layer (Sapolsky, 2000). The dentate gyrus is one of the sites of neurogenesis in the adult brain and one of the brain regions thought to play a role in the formation of new memories. At this level, the glutamatergic system modulates the growth of neurons' dendrites to form neuronal nets that translate salient stimuli in permanent or semipermanent informative biological structures, thanks to long-term potentiation (LTP). During depressive states, the chronic activation of the system may be responsible for neuronal death and the subsequent decrease in the hippocampal volume. We must remember here that neuronal systems are involved in complex co-regulation: in the hippocampus, the firing of glutamate neurons is regulated though interplay with the serotoninergic (5-HT2, 5-HT4 and 5-HT5 receptors) and noradrenergic ($\alpha 1$ receptor) systems (Drago *et al*., 2011). Consistent with the role of glutamate in MDD pathogenesis, it has been well known that compounds which target the glutamatergic system have an antidepressant effect since the 1950s, when D-cycloserine, a partial agonist at the NMDA receptor glycine site used as an antituberculosis drug, was reported to have mood-elevating effects (Manji *et al*., 2003). The glutamatergic modulators lamotrigine and riluzole, both inhibitors of glutamate release, show antidepressant properties too.

Particular attention has been given to ketamine, which acts through inhibition of NMDA receptors, because it reverses the behavioural and physiological alterations induced by chronic mild stress in rats and has been proven to be an antidepressant in humans (Drago *et al*., 2011). In patients suffering from TRD, ketamine shows rapid onset and marked antidepressant action (response rate of 71% after 24 hours), but the antidepressant effect lasts only for a few days (Zarate *et al*., 2010). The mechanism of the ketamine antidepressant effect has not been clarified as yet, but it has recently been proposed that both NMDA antagonism and AMPA receptor activation are involved. The NMDA receptors have a slower and more prolonged postsynaptic current than the AMPA receptors, which show the property of inducing a more rapid dissociation of glutamate, and the antidepressant effect probably results from the 'correct' balance of NMDA and AMPA receptor activity in definite brain areas. In any case, the antidepressant effect of glutamatergic substances may be partially due to monoaminergic mechanisms: downregulation of the adrenergic receptors and enhancement of the serotoninergic function are associated with the administration of glutamatergic antidepressant substances. Thus chronic treatment with antidepressants causes a reduction of glutamate release (Drago *et al.*, 2011). The reported findings also lead to the hypothesis that the NMDA receptor complex may mediate the delayed therapeutic effects of traditional monoaminergic-based antidepressants, suggesting that new antidepressants directly targeting the glutamatergic system may show rapid clinical effects and be effective in TRD.

Despite the relevance of the glutamatergic system in MDD and antidepressant mechanisms of action, glutamatergic genes have been only marginally studied until now as predictors of antidepressant efficacy. The most investigated gene as a predictor of response is GRIK4 (glutamate receptor, ionotropic, kainate 4), which codes for glutamate kainate receptors responsible for postsynaptic inhibitory neurotransmission, but results are scant and inconsistent. Interestingly, other genes may be predictors of treatment-emergent suicidal ideation (GRIK2 and glutamate receptor ionotrophic AMPA 3 or GRIA3) or sexual dysfunction (GRIK2, GRIA1, GRIA3 and glutamate receptor ionotropic N-methyl-D-aspartate 3A or GRIN3A), but confirmations are needed (Porcelli *et al.*, 2011c). These genes all code for subunits of glutamate ionotropic receptors, and, despite their key role, they represent only the first step in the glutamatergic molecular cascade. A number of interrelated genes are still to be investigated. An interesting line of research points toward the KCNK2 (potassium channel subfamily K member 2) gene, which codes for a two-pore-domain potassium channel involved in the regulation of excitability and the resting potentials of neurons. The opening of these channels may be inhibited by stimulation of the metabotropic glutamate receptors, mGluR1 and mGluR5. KCNK2 is expressed in brain areas implicated in MDD, including the prefrontal cortex, hippocampus and other limbic structures. Animal models further suggest its involvement in the pathophysiology of MDD and in antidepressant response: KCNK2 KO mice show increased efficacy of 5-HT neurotransmission, resistance to depression and a substantially reduced elevation of corticosterone levels under stress. Moreover, KCNK2 KO mice show behaviour similar to that of naïve animals under antidepressant treatment (Heurteaux *et al.*, 2006), suggesting that the action of antidepressants may partly depend on KCNK2 inhibition. Given these promising preclinical data, the effect of this gene on antidepressant response has been studied in the largest clinical trial to include unipolar depressed patients performed to date (the Sequenced Treatment Alternatives to Relieve Depression or STAR*D study) (Perlis *et al.*, 2008). Several SNPs within the KCNK2 gene were found to be predictors of nonremission after first- and second-line treatments, suggesting that the gene plays a role in TRD only. Interestingly, genotypes found to be associated with antidepressant response (at rs10494996, rs2841608 and rs2841616) showed higher frequency in subjects with basal ganglia activity potentiated to gain, suggesting that KCNK2 may be involved in motivation and anhedonia (Porcelli *et al.*, 2011c). Among the molecular players interrelated with glutamate receptors, another promising gene is RGS4 (regulator of G protein signalling 4), a member of a family of regulatory molecules that act as GTPase-activating proteins (GAPs) for G alpha subunits. RGS4 modulates several G protein-coupled receptors that have been suggested to play a major role in the treatment of MDD: metabotropic glutamate, serotonin and dopamine receptors. In animal models, electroconvulsive shocks induced subtype-, time- and region-specific alteration of RGS proteins (Gold *et al.*, 2002). Furthermore, in healthy subjects the A allele at rs951436 was associated with hypofunctionality in working memory tasks and delayed information processing, both of which are altered in affective disorders (Buckholtz *et al.*, 2007). Despite these findings, preliminary results did not demonstrate any effect of rs951436 on either ECT response in TRD or the risk of TRD (Huuhka *et al.*, 2008b). Nevertheless, only one polymorphism has been studied so far and the impact on specific symptom clusters (particularly cognitive dysfunction) has not been investigated.

Despite these preliminary results, a number of other genes acting in the metabolic pathway of glutamate have not yet been investigated (Drago *et al.*, 2011), leaving undisclosed potential key genetic variants affecting the great interindividual variability observed in antidepressant efficacy. The antidepressant efficacy of ketamine in TRD suggests that targeting the glutamatergic system may be a promising way of restoring the biological alterations made by MDD, acting on an alternative molecular pathway when the monoaminergic system is 'poorly responsive'.

Growth factors and inflammation: neuroplasticity in MDD and antidepressant response

Neurotrophic factors were first characterized as regulating neural growth and differentiation during development, but are now known to be potent regulators of plasticity and survival of neurons and glia during adulthood. Accordingly, some recent findings have revealed that newborn neurons exist in the mature brains of mammals, humans included. A role for neuronal plasticity in affective disorders was hypothesized through the neurotrophin hypothesis of depression (Porcelli *et al.*, 2011a), which states that a deficiency in neurotrophic support may contribute to hippocampal pathology during MDD and that antidepressant treatments may reverse this deficiency, contributing to clinical response. Indeed, a diminished volume of specific brain areas in MDD (the hippocampus, left anterior cingulate gyrus, subgenual region, area 9 (dorsolateral cortex), area 10/47 (rostral orbital cortex) and area 47 (caudal orbital cortex)) can be reversed by antidepressant drugs (Porcelli *et al.*, 2011a). Given the wide use of the terms 'synaptic plasticity' and 'neuroplasticity', we shall clarify that the former refers to the cellular process that results in lasting changes in the efficacy of neurotransmission, while the latter is a broader term that includes changes in intracellular signalling cascades and gene regulation, modifications of synaptic number and strength, modelling of axonal and dendritic architecture, variations in neurotransmitter release and, in some areas of the CNS, neurogenesis. In MDD, the defective production of neuro-trophic factors has been hypothesized to be due to the interplay of several factors: imbalance in monoamine and glutamatergic neurotransmission and dysfunction of the hypothalamic–pituitary–adrenal (HPA) axis (Figure 3.1). Indeed, atrophy of CA3 pyramidal neurons was demonstrated after exposure to high levels of glucocorticoids, and both type I (mineralocorti-coid receptor or MR) and type II (glucocorticoid receptor or GR) corticosteroid receptors are expressed in the hippocampus (Manji *et al.*, 2003). In this brain region, the activation of type II receptors causes increased calcium currents and enhanced responses to excitatory amino acids. Thus, very high levels of type II receptor activation lead to increased NMDA receptor throughput, which could predispose to neurotoxicity. Never-theless, the hyperactivity of the HPA axis *per se* does not explain the reduction in BDNF (brain-derived neurotrophic fac-tor, a member of the neurotrophin family of growth factors) levels, since a high dose of glucocorticoid is not enough to decrease BDNF and adrenalectomy does not block the effect of stress. On the other hand, the inflammatory theory of depres-sion, which is highly interrelated with the neurotrophin one, posits that an imbalance in the immune mediators is involved in the pathogenesis of depressive symptoms. Anyone who has ever caught the flu knows that being sick involves ignoring food and beverages and losing interest in the physical and social environment, which is reminiscent of what happens during MDD. Proinflammatory cytokines cause various clinical aspects of depression, including hyperactivity of the HPA, dis-turbed 5-HT metabolism and neurovegetative symptoms. The inflammatory hypothesis is supported by the finding of eleva-tions in proinflammatory cytokines and other inflammation-related proteins in the plasma and cerebrospinal fluid (CSF) of MDD subjects, as well as in post-mortem brain, while antide-pressants can lead to a normalization of these parameters (Porcelli *et al.*, 2011a). Among the regulators of inflammatory cytokines, the purinergic receptor P2X, ligand-gated ion channel 7 (P2RX7) acts as a ligand-gated ion channel and mediates the release of proinflammatory cytokines such as interleukin-1β, which is a key mediator in chronic inflammation, neurodegeneration and chronic pain. P2X7 receptor-deficient mice show a substantially attenuated inflammatory response (Chessell et al., 2005). Although the expression of this nuclear receptor is still uncertain in neurons, it is demonstrated in cells from haematopoietic lineages and epithelial and endothelial cells, and its activation can mediate and/or enhance neurotransmitter release (e.g. glutamate) and may affect neuronal plasticity and neuronal cell death. Thus, P2X7 receptors may function as mediators between the immune and the nervous system and play a role in both neurodegenerative and psychiatric disorders. Two functional polymorphisms identified within the P2X7 gene seem to increase the risk of a familial mood disorder and time spent ill, but preliminary data have not demonstrated any association between these SNPs and the risk of TRD or treatment (ECT or SSRI) response (Viikki et al., 2011a). Further investigation is needed to clarify the contribution of P2X7 and other inflammatory genes to the antidepressant response and particularly TRD.

Consistent with the role of neuroplasticity in MDD pathogenesis, chronic, although not acute, antidepressant treatment (Jacobs et al., 2000) and electroconvulsive seizure (Segi-Nishida, 2011) increase the expression of BDNF and neurogenesis of dentate gyrus granule cells. BDNF and the molecular players acting within its signalling cascade are considered key mediators of neuroplasticity and thus promising candidates for pharmacogenetic studies and targets for new antidepressant drugs. Indeed, neurotrophins support the differentiation and survival of neurons, as well as the modulation of synaptic transmission and synaptic plasticity. They bind to and activate both specific receptor tyrosine kinases belonging to the Trk family of receptors and the pan-neurotrophin receptor P75. Increasing evidence suggests that neurotrophic factors inhibit cell-death cascades by activating the mitogen-activated protein (MAP) kinase signalling pathway and the phosphotidylinositol-3 kinase/Akt pathway (Figure 3.1). The activation of MAP kinase signalling cascades results in an increased expression of the antiapoptotic protein bcl-2, which probably represents one of the main mechanisms of cell-survival promotion (Manji *et al*., 2003). Decreased expression of BDNF and members of its signalling pathway (TrkB and cAMP response element-binding protein or CREB) have been demonstrated in the post-mortem prefrontal cortex and hippocampus of both suicide victims and stressed rats (Yu & Chen, 2011). In any case, the role of BDNF signalling in MDD pathogenesis and antidepressant response cannot be simply imputed to a reduction of its expression. Indeed, BDNF overexpression into dopaminergic areas (the ventral tegmental area and the nucleus accumbens) could lead to a hyperstimulation of dopaminergic neurons, which would eventually be detrimental for mood (Porcelli *et al*., 2011a). The BDNF gene consists of four 5′ noncoding exons (I–IV), each with a separate promotor, and one 3′ exon (exon-V) encoding the mature BDNF protein. Chronic administration of antidepressants leads to brain-region-specific upregulation of specific BDNF alternative splicing products, suggesting that genetic variants affecting the regulation of gene expression may impact on antidepressant efficacy. The SNP rs6265 (196G/A), which results in a valine to methionine (V66M) substitution, has gained particular attention for its functional effect. Indeed, the Met allele has been associated with low depolarization-induced secretion of BDNF and BDNF failure in localizing into secretory granules or synapses (Egan *et al*., 2003). Hippocampal volume has been found to be decreased in healthy volunteers and depressed patients carrying the Met allele (Scharinger *et al*., 2011). At a functional level, the Met allele was associated with poorer episodic memory, abnormal hippocampal activation assayed with fMRI and lower hippocampal n-acetyl aspartate (NAA), assayed with MRI spectroscopy (Egan *et al*., 2003). Increasing evidence from pharmacogenetic studies supports a role for rs6265 in antidepressant response, even if there is still controversy about whether allele or genotype should be considered the risk factor in both TRD and non-TRD (Porcelli *et al*.,

2011c). These contradictory findings are a typical example of the difficulty of translating hypotheses suggested by preclinical data and imaging studies into pharmacogenetic confirmations. Several confounding factors probably lie behind this issue (see the 'Conclusions' section), among which we should remember the inadequate genetic coverage. Indeed, the available results mainly derive from studies focused on a single SNP harboured by a candidate gene, without any consideration of the possible modulating effect caused by other variants within the same gene or related genes. As a matter of fact, recently two BDNF SNPs other than rs6265 (rs10501087 and rs1491850) (Kocabas *et al.*, 2011) and an interaction between rs6265 and rs6295 (5-HT1A gene) (Anttila *et al.*, 2007a) were identified as possible risk factors for TRD.

Within the BDNF molecular pathway, the literature provides some evidence of involvement in antidepressant response of the gene CREB1, which encodes a transcription factor that is a member of the leucine zipper family of DNA-binding proteins. Several growth factors and stress signals stimulate CREB-mediated transcription by promoting the phosphorylation of CREB at Ser133 by means of various cellular kinases. In turn, CREB binds to specific DNA sequences called cAMP response elements (CREs) and regulates gene expression. Induction of BDNF is at least partly mediated by CREB. In humans, alterations in CREB have been associated with the pathophysiology of depression and suicide (Dwivedi *et al.*, 2003), as well as the mechanism of antidepressant action and response. Indeed, increased CREB levels in rodent models result in antidepressant-like behaviours, and studies on both humans and rodents have shown that CREB is upregulated by chronic antidepressant treatment (Blendy, 2006). Hence, it could be hypothesized that specific variants within CREB1 might be related to a lower likelihood of recovery from MDD, possibly through a differential modulation of gene expression and activation. Furthermore, CREB1 lies in a region of chromosome 2 (q33–q35) that has been associated with the risk of MDD in women and whose G(−656)A variant has been found to modulate the development of the disease in women, through selective alteration of CREB1 promoter activity by female gonadal steroids in noradrenergic neuronal cells (Serretti *et al.*, 2011a). Several SNPs within this gene have been studied with regard to both the risk of MDD and antidepressant response, with some positive results found for the former but not for the latter (Porcelli *et al.*, 2011c). Despite these negative results, the possible role of this gene in antidepressant response has recently been brought into question once again, in regard to TRD alone. Indeed, subjects carrying the A allele at rs7569963, the AA haplotype at rs2253206–rs7569963 and the AC haloptype at rs7569963–rs4675690 have been found to have increased risk of developing TRD (Serretti *et al.*, 2011a). Furthermore, a cytosine deletion within the gene may be a predictor of reduced TRD risk (Wilkie *et al.*, 2007). The role of CREB1 in the modulation of antidepressant response may thus become clearer over repeated trials, suggesting an effect that is quite independent of the specific drug, since it acts at a deeper level in the cascade of events related to antidepressant response.

The genes whose transcription is regulated by CREB include vascular endothelial growth factor (VEGF), which was first characterized (and named) for its role in vascular permeability and was later described as a potent endothelial cell mitogen and survival factor. Recently, it has been found to play roles that move beyond the vascular system. Indeed, aside from regulating endothelial cells and blood vessel formation/permeability, a role as a true neurotrophic factor has been hypothesized. In the hippocampus, neural progenitors are found proliferating in dense clusters associated with the vasculature, and one-third of them are immunopositive for markers of endothelial cells. Thus, neuronal cell proliferation may be promoted indirectly by VEGF, through the stimulation of endothelial cell proliferation, which in turn induces neural progenitor cell division. The alternative – and no less probable – hypothesis is that VEGF exerts a direct mitogenic effect on neural progenitors. Indeed, recent studies demonstrate that VEGF signalling through Flk-1 (foetal liver kinase, one of the two high-affinity VEGF receptors) increases proliferation of neuronal progenitors, stimulates adult neurogenesis *in vitro* and *in vivo* and promotes neurite outgrowth (Warner-Schmidt & Duman, 2008). Consistent with the neurotrophin hypothesis of depression, several classes of antidepressant and electroconvulsive seizure increase VEGF expression in rat hippocampus (Segi-Nishida, 2011), and in humans ECT has been associated with an increase in VEGF serum concentration (Minelli *et al.*, 2011). Similarly, stress reduces VEGF expression in the same region (Warner-Schmidt & Duman, 2008). Despite it seeming a good candidate gene, VEGF is as yet poorly studied in the field of antidepressant pharmacogenetics, and several markers (rs1570360, rs2010963, rs25648, rs833069, rs3025010, rs3025033 and rs3025039) have provided negative results. rs699947 (2578 C/A) is still the only known variant with a possible impact on the risk of TRD (Viikki *et al.*, 2010a). Interestingly, this polymorphism has been associated with VEGF expression (Steffensen *et al.*, 2010) and the risk of neurodegenerative diseases (Del Bo *et al.*, 2005), suggesting the need for further investigation to better dissect its role in MDD, and TRD in particular.

Antidepressant pharmacokinetics

Aside from genetic variants involved in antidepressant pharmacodynamics, polymorphisms located within key genes involved in antidepressant metabolism and clearance may also play a relevant role in the interindividual difference observed in treatment efficacy. The genes coding for the cytochrome P450 (CYP) isoenzymes and P-glycoprotein (P-gp) (MDR1 or ABCB1) have been particular targets of investigation, since their products are mainly responsible for antidepressant transport and metabolism (Porcelli *et al.*, 2011c).

Cytochrome P450 genes

The CYP superfamily is the major enzyme class responsible for the oxidation and reduction of numerous organic substrates, with over 50 isoenzymes known to date (http://www.cypalleles.ki.se).

The key role of these enzymes in drug metabolism and the highly polymorphic nature of their coding genes make them an interesting subject for pharmacogenetics. Their activity level is usually described by a conventional nomenclature, although it does not exactly reflect their metabolic status since it doesn't take into account that some alleles are only partially active, some show different activities depending on the drug metabolized and several substances can induce or inhibit CYP activity (Porcelli *et al.*, 2011d). According to this classification, the wild-type genotype or extensive metabolizer (EM) is characterized by the presence of two active alleles, while the intermediate metabolizer (IM) is characterized by the presence of one wild-type allele plus a partially or totally defective allele. The IM is expected to be found between the EMs and the poor metabolizers (PMs). PMs show a combination of two partially or totally defective alleles. Finally, the ultrarapid metabolizer (UM) category exists only for CYP2D6 and is usually linked to multiple copies of the *1 or *2A allele (Porcelli *et al.*, 2011d). The most relevant CYP isoforms in antidepressant metabolism are CYP2D6, CYP2C19, CYP2C9, CYP1A2 and CYP2B6. Some evidence suggests that CYP2D6 PM status may be associated with increased risk of drug-related adverse events, while CYP2D6 EM – or, for venlafaxine, CYP2D6 PM status – may predict nonresponse and the risk of suicide (Porcelli *et al.*, 2011d). Nevertheless, the available studies have mainly not found any association between CYP genotype or phenotype and antidepressant response, while these genes can have an impact on tolerance to both tricyclic antidepressants (TCAs) and venlafaxine (Porcelli *et al.*, 2011d). There is therefore no evidence to date to support the use of CYP genotyping tests, such as the already commercialized AmpliChip™ test, in order to identify TRD patients.

P-glycoprotein (MDR1 or ABCB1)

P-gp, a member of the superfamily of ATP-binding cassette (ABC) transporter proteins, is an ATP-dependent drug efflux pump for xenobiotic compounds, which decreases drug accumulation in multidrug-resistant cells and limits uptake of some lipophilic drugs into key organs such as the brain (Porcelli *et al.*, 2011c). The transporter is widely expressed in human tissues, not only at the level of organs involved in the catabolism and the elimination of drugs but also in the luminal membranes of endothelial cells of the blood–brain barrier. Animal studies show that a wide variety of structurally unrelated drugs are efficaciously carried out of the brain by P-gp activity, among which are a long list of antidepressants (with some exceptions, such as fluoxetine and bupropion) (Porcelli *et al.*, 2011c). On the other hand, some antidepressants may affect P-gp activity; for example, nefazodone inhibits P-gp function, while St John's wort and venlafaxine enhance it (Porcelli *et al.*, 2011c). ABC transporters have been implicated in resistance to pharmacotherapy, most notably in oncology, where the expression of these efflux pumps by cancer cells can confer resistance to chemotherapy (O'Brien *et al.*, 2011). Over 50 functional SNPs have been identified within the ABCB1 gene to date, and several studies have demonstrated that they can impact on P-gp expression and function in humans, and therefore influence the pharmacokinetics of various drugs, including antidepressants (O'Brien *et al.*, 2011). The most studied polymorphisms are the functional SNPs rs2032582 and rs1045642, but their association with antidepressant efficacy is still controversial (Porcelli *et al.*, 2011c). rs2232583 may be involved in resistance to antidepressant treatment: the TT genotype has been hypothesized to increase drug export from the brain, requiring dose adjustment or switching to a drug that is not a substrate of P-gp (Rosenhagen & Uhr, 2010; Uhr *et al.*, 2008).

Conclusions

A high number of pharmacokinetic and pharmacodynamic genes may contribute to the clinical outcome of antidepressant treatments, explaining the hypothesized 50% variance in response ascribed to genetic factors. The variance in antidepressant response due to a single gene is estimated to be low (e.g. 3.2% for 5-HTTLPR (Serretti *et al.*, 2011c)), so future pharmacogenetic tests will likely include multiple loci. Nonetheless, antidepressant pharmacogenetic studies have so far provided poorly replicated and often contradictory results. A possible explanation for this discouraging fact concerns the main phenotype investigated so far: MDD itself. The standard criteria for the diagnosis of MDD are probably not discriminative enough to identify a homogeneous group of patients. In fact, it has been hypothesized that MDD represents a common final phenotype of various different pathophysiological mechanisms. Therefore, in recent years researchers have tried to identify more homogeneous subgroups of patients characterized by common features (endophenotypes, such as MDD with psychotic features or TRD) in order to obtain more informative pharmacogenetic results. Despite the usefulness of focusing on the TRD endophenotype (the current response and remission rates are around 47 and 33%, respectively (Trivedi *et al.*, 2006)), it is still poorly studied in the field of pharmacogenetics. So far, the most promising genes for association with TRD seem to be SLC6A4, 5-HTR1A, COMT, BDNF and CREB1 (for an overview of pharmacogenetic results concerning TRD, see Table 3.1), but much work is still needed in order to translate findings into clinical recommendations. Nonetheless, the results reached thanks to pharmacogenetic research in other fields of medicine, especially oncology (Paik *et al.*, 2006; Slodkowska & Ross, 2009), allow for cautious optimism within psychiatry.

In order to reach our objectives, the methodological limitations of previous pharmacogenetic studies should be carefully considered, since they probably explain the low number of confirmed results and the high rate of contradictory findings. We must keep in mind that the replication of pharmacogenetic results is necessary, given the high risk of false-positive findings using both the candidate gene approach and GWAS (Sullivan, 2007). Among the main methodological limitations are a lack of consideration of the heterogeneity of many clinical samples, with regard to not only different subtypes of MDD but

Table 3.1 Summary of pharmacogenetic studies in treatment-resistant depression (TRD) samples

Gene	Polymorphism	Study	Treatment	Result	Sample size, ethnicity
SLC4A6	5-HTTLPR	Malaguti et al. (2011)	rMTS augmentation during pharmacotherapy	No association	90 Caucasian
		Reimherr et al. (2010)	Sertraline + atomoxetine	SS ↑ remission	50 Caucasian subsample
		Kishida et al. (2007)	Mainly medication-free for at least 2 weeks	No different allele/ genotype frequency between cases and controls	119 patients 141 healthy controls Caucasian
		Bocchio-Chiavetto et al. (2008)	rMTS augmentation during pharmacotherapy	L/L ↑ response	36 Caucasian
		Zanardi et al. (2007)	rMTS augmentation during pharmacotherapy	L ↑ response	47 TRD 52 non-TRD Caucasian
5-HTTLPR and rs25531		Bonvicini et al. (2010)	Naturalistic pharmacotherapy	L allele, L_A, $L_A L_A$ genotype, higher frequency in controls	310 patients 284 healthy controls Caucasian
5-HTTLPR and VNTR (STin2)		Kishida et al. (2007)	Mainly medication-free for at least 2 weeks	No association	119 patients 141 healthy controls Caucasian

Gene	SNP	Reference	Treatment	Result	Sample
5-HTR1A	rs6295 (1019 C > G)	Brent et al. (2010)	SSRIs	No association	176 SSRI-resistant (adolescents) Caucasian
		Anttila et al. (2007b)	ECT	GG genotype + GA +AA at rs6265 (BDNF) ↑ risk of TRD	119 patients 392 healthy controls Caucasian
		Noro et al. (2010)	Naturalistic pharmacotherapy	C allele trend of association with TRD	75 TRD 117 nonresponders 180 nonremitters Caucasian
		Zanardi et al. (2007)	rMTS augmentation during pharmacotherapy	CC genotype ↑ response	47 TRD 52 non-TRD Caucasian
		Malaguti et al. (2011)	rMTS augmentation during pharmacotherapy	CC genotype ↑ response	90 Caucasian
		Brent et al. (2010)	SSRIs	No association	176 SSRI-resistant (adolescents) Caucasian
	rs6295 and six other SNPs	Levin et al. (2007)	SSRIs	No association	33 SSRI nonresponders 100 SSRI responders 100 healthy controls Mixed ethnicity

(Continued)

Table 3.1 (Continued)

Gene	Polymorphism	Study	Treatment	Result	Sample size, ethnicity
5-HTR2A	rs7997012	Noro et al. (2010)	Naturalistic pharmacotherapy	A allele associated with TRD (not survived after Bonferroni correction)	75 TRD 117 nonresponders 180 nonremitters Caucasian
	rs7997012 and rs6311	Viikki et al. (2011b)	ECT and SSRIs	GA genotype at rs7997012 and TT at rs6311 ↑ response	119 TRD 99 non-TRD Caucasian
	rs6313, rs6311, rs2070040 and rs6314	Brent et al. (2010)	SSRIs	No association	176 SSRI-resistant (adolescents) Caucasian
TPH1	rs1800532 (218A/C)	Viikki et al. (2010b)	ECT and SSRIs	CC genotype ↑ frequency in TRD compared to non-TRD and ↓ response	119 TRD 98 non-TRD 395 healthy controls Caucasian
		Anttila et al. (2007b)	ECT	CC genotype in combination with the T allele at C825T *GNB3* ↑ risk to be in the TRD group	119 patients 398 healthy controls Caucasian

Gene	Polymorphism	Study	Treatment	Result	Sample
	rs1800532, rs4757610 and rs623580	Brent et al. (2010)	SSRIs	No association	176 SSRI-resistant (adolescents) Caucasian
TPH2	rs1386494 and rs1843809	Anttila et al. (2009)	ECT	rs1386494 A/A genotype ↑ improvement, no effect of rs1843809	119 patients 385 controls Caucasian
	G1463A	Zhang et al. (2005)	No current MD	A allele associated with SSRI-non response	87 unipolar MD 60 bipolar MD 219 controls Mixed
	G1463A, C1487G and T1578G	Garriock et al. (2005)	Not reported	No difference in frequency between cases and controls	91 TRD 99 non-TRD 186 healthy controls Mixed
COMT	rs4680	Domschke et al. (2010)	ECT	Val (G) and Val/Val ↑ response	104 Caucasian
		Anttila et al. (2008)	ECT	Val/Val ↑ response	119 Caucasian
		Malaguti et al. (2011)	rMTS augmentation during pharmacotherapy	No association	90 Caucasian
	rs4680 and DRD2 rs6277 (C957T)	Huuhka et al. (2008a)	ECT	rs6277 TT + rs4680 Met/ Met ↓ remission	118 383 healthy controls Caucasian

(Continued)

Table 3.1 (Continued)

Gene	Polymorphism	Study	Treatment	Result	Sample size, ethnicity
	rs2075507, rs737865, rs6269, rs4633, rs4818, rs4680 and rs165599	Kocabas et al. (2010)	Naturalistic pharmacotherapy	rs2075507 G and G/G and rs165599 C associated with TRD	105 TRD 294 nonresponders 240 nonremitters Caucasian
	rs4680, rs2075507, rs737865, rs6269, rs4633, rs4818 and rs165599	Schosser et al. (2011)	Naturalistic pharmacotherapy	rs2075507, rs737865 and rs6269 associated with suicide risk only in nonresponders	250 Caucasian
MAOA	Promoter VNTR	Aklillu et al. (2009)	Mainly free from antidepressants	Short alleles associated with atypical MD in TRD women	118 Caucasian
		Brent et al. (2010)	SSRIs	No association	176 SSRI-resistant (adolescents) Caucasian
CREB1	rs2709376, rs2253206, rs7569963, rs7594560 and rs4675690	Serretti et al. (2011b)	Naturalistic pharmacotherapy	rs7569963 A allele and rs2253206/rs7569963 AA haplotype associated with TRD	71 TRD 63 responders 20 remitters 76 healthy controls Caucasian

	Polymorphism	Reference	Treatment	Finding	N
CREBBP	Intron 8 C deletion	Wilkie et al. (2007)	Naturalistic pharmacotherapy	C deletion nonsignificantly more frequent in remitters and responders after second switch	163 Caucasian
	T651 C	Wilkie et al. (2007)	Naturalistic pharmacotherapy	No association	163 Caucasian
BDNF	rs6265 (196 A > G)	Bocchio-Chiavetto et al. (2008)	rTMS augmentation during pharmacotherapy	Val/Val ↑ response	36 Caucasian
		Brent et al. (2010)	SSRIs	No association	176 SSRI-resistant (adolescents) Caucasian
		Wilkie et al. (2007)	Naturalistic pharmacotherapy	No association	163 Caucasian
	rs6265, rs10501087 and rs1491850	Kocabas et al. (2011)	Naturalistic pharmacotherapy	rs6265 Val, rs10501087 T and rs1491850 T alleles associated with the risk of TRD	75 TRD 117 nonresponders 180 nonremitters Caucasian
	rs6265 and C270T	Huuhka et al. (2007)	ECT	No association	119 Caucasian

(Continued)

Table 3.1 (Continued)

Gene	Polymorphism	Study	Treatment	Result	Sample size, ethnicity
VEGF	rs699947 (2578 C/A)	Viikki et al. (2010a)	ECT and SSRIs	CC genotype associated with TRD but not with ECT response	119 TRD 98 non-TRD 395 healthy controls Caucasian
ACE 1	Insertion/deletion within intron 16	Stewart et al. (2009)	ECT	No association	119 TRD 392 healthy controls Caucasian
P2RX7	rs2230912 and rs208294	Viikki et al. (2011a)	ECT and SSRIs	No association	119 TRD 98 non-TRD 382 healthy controls Caucasian
ABCB1	rs2232583	Rosenhagen et al. (2010)	Various antidepressants	TT genotype associated with TRD	2 case reports
RGS4	rs951436	Huuhka et al. (2008b)	ECT	No association	119 TRD 384 healthy controls Caucasian

Gene	SNP(s)	Study	Treatment	Result	Sample
APOE	rs429358 and rs7412 (alleles ε3, ε2 and ε4)	Huuhka et al. (2005)	ECT	No association with response, in women ε2 may play a protective role in cognition	119 TRD 398 healthy controls Caucasian
PTGS2	rs4648276, rs2066826 and rs689466	Serretti et al. (2011b)	Naturalistic pharmacotherapy	No association	81 TRD 77 responders 27 remitters Caucasian
DTNBP1	rs760761 and rs2619522	Kokobas et al. (2011)	Naturalistic pharmacotherapy	No association	75 TRD 117 nonresponders 180 nonremitters Caucasian
KCNK2	rs10779646, rs17546779, rs2841608, rs2841616, rs7549184 and rs10494996	Perlis et al. (2008)	Mixed-drug therapy or cognitive therapy	Association with remission after second or third antidepressant trial	751 patients in second trial 225 patients in third trial Mixed
GNB3	rs5443 (C825T)	Wilkie et al. (2007)	Naturalistic pharmacotherapy	TT genotype associated with nonresponse and nonremission after second switch	163 Caucasian

also the common use of different treatments and the inclusion of individuals with different ethnic origins. The number of previous depressive episodes and the age at onset should also be considered as stratification factors, since subjects with a single-episode history or late onset likely have a lower genetic loading (Tsuang, 1990). Furthermore, the symptomatology features and the psychological profile may help to define more homogeneous subgroups of patients with more homogeneous determinants, as suggested by several authors (Baffa *et al.*, 2010; Mandelli *et al.*, 2010). This matter is related to the complex nature of MDD and antidepressant response, which results from the interaction of genetic, intrinsic nongenetic (e.g. clinical, sociodemographic and psychological determinants) and environmental factors. Thus, statistical analysis must also become more complex, through GWAS, pathway-analysis and gene–environment interaction studies. These new perspectives on pharmacogenetics have begun to become real applications in recent years, even if technical (e.g. low genetic coverage) or design (e.g. no side-effect or compliance assessment) defects are common limitations of past, and sometimes also recent, studies. Today the reported and other issues are better known; indeed, the relevance of genetic confounding factors such as the so-called 'flip-flop' phenomenon, *de novo* mutations and epigenetic modifications is emerging.

The flip-flop phenomenon is the result of the interaction of multiple loci and environmental effects in determining susceptibility to complex diseases such as MDD, which may lead to ambiguous results. For example, flip-flop associations can be caused by investigation of a noncausal variant in LD (linkage disequilibrium) using a genuine causal variant. With regard to this issue, notable difference in LD across populations have been found (e.g. for the COMT gene), and less obviously, sampling variation can lead to variations in observed LD patterns. For this reason, markers in weak LD with each other (e.g. $r^2 < 0.3$) may need to be considered carefully (Lin *et al.*, 2007).

The idea that *de novo* mutations and epigenetic modifications can affect a clinical phenotype is a recent one, so they are still poorly investigated. Nonetheless, preliminary findings suggest that epigenetic mechanisms may play a relevant role in regulating the expression of key genes during antidepressant treatment (Mamdani *et al.*, 2011). On the other hand, the effect of *de novo* (point substitutions or single-nucleotide variants and small insertions or deletions) and recurrent mutations has recently been hypothesized to be a further cause of poor replication of genetic findings in psychiatry (Xu *et al.*, 2008). The availability of next-generation whole-genome or whole-exome sequencing allows the study of *de novo* mutations in a systematic genome-wide manner, enabling us to clarify their role in MDD and thus TRD.

Our increasing knowledge of the limits that have affected antidepressant pharmacogenetic studies until now, together with technological improvement, is gradually expected to allow interesting advances to be made. Multiple-loci genotyping tests are anticipated to provide cost-effective information under given indications (e.g. in patients at higher risk of TRD or drug-related adverse events) and for the recurrent nature of MDD (Serretti *et al.*, 2011c). Given this assumption, there is great hope that pharmacogenomics will offer personalized treatments based on genetic profiles of response/side effects, leading to a radical improvement of prognosis in MDD and TRD, and in other common and disabling psychiatric diseases.

References

Aklillu, E., Karlsson, S., Zachrisson, O. O. *et al.* (2009) Association of MAOA gene functional promoter polymorphism with CSF dopamine turnover and atypical depression. *Pharmacogen. Gen.*, **19**(4), 267–275.

Albert, P. R. & Francois, B. L. (2010) Modifying 5-HT1A receptor gene expression as a new target for antidepressant therapy. *Front. Neurosci.*, **4**, 35.

Anttila, S., Huuhka, K., Huuhka, M. *et al.* (2007a) Interaction between 5-HT1A and BDNF genotypes increases the risk of treatment-resistant depression. *J. Neural. Transm.*, **114**(8), 1065–1068.

Anttila, S., Huuhka, K., Huuhka, M. *et al.* (2007b) Interaction between TPH1 and GNB3 genotypes and electroconvulsive therapy in major depression. *J. Neural. Transm.*, **114**(4), 461–468.

Anttila, S., Huuhka, K., Huuhka, M. *et al.* (2008) Catechol-O-methyltransferase (COMT) polymorphisms predict treatment response in electroconvulsive therapy. *Pharmacogen. J.*, **8**(2), 113–116.

Anttila, S., Viikki, M., Huuhka, K. *et al.* (2009) TPH2 polymorphisms may modify clinical picture in treatment-resistant depression. *Neurosci. Lett.*, **464**(1), 43–46.

Baffa, A., Hohoff, C., Baune, B. T. *et al.* (2010) Norepinephrine and serotonin transporter genes: impact on treatment response in depression. *Neuropsychobiol.*, **62**(2), 121–131.

Blendy, J. A. (2006) The role of CREB in depression and antidepressant treatment. *Biol. Psychiatry*, **59**(12), 1144–1150.

Bocchio-Chiavetto, L., Miniussi, C., Zanardini, R. *et al.* (2008) 5-HTTLPR and BDNF Val66Met polymorphisms and response to rTMS treatment in drug resistant depression. *Neurosci. Lett.*, **437**(2), 130–134.

Bonvicini, C., Minelli, A., Scassellati, C. *et al.* (2010) Serotonin transporter gene polymorphisms and treatment-resistant depression. *Prog. Neuropsychopharmacol. Biol. Psychiatry*, **34**(6), 934–939.

Brent, D., Melhem, N., Ferrell, R. *et al.* (2010) Association of FKBP5 polymorphisms with suicidal events in the Treatment of Resistant Depression in Adolescents (TORDIA) study. *Am. J. Psychiatry*, **167**(2), 190–197.

Buckholtz, J. W., Meyer-Lindenberg, A., Honea, R. A. *et al.* (2007) Allelic variation in RGS4 impacts functional and structural connectivity in the human brain. *J. Neurosci.*, **27**(7), 1584–1593.

Chessell, I. P., Hatcher, J. P., Bountra, C. *et al.* (2005) Disruption of the P2X7 purinoceptor gene abolishes chronic inflammatory and neuropathic pain. *Pain*, **114**(3), 386–396.

Del Bo, R., Scarlato, M., Ghezzi, S. *et al.* (2005) Vascular endothelial growth factor gene variability is associated with increased risk for AD. *Ann. Neurology*, **57**(3), 373–380.

Dhaenen, H. (2001) Imaging the serotonergic system in depression. *Eur. Arch. Psychiatry Clin. Neurosci.*, **251**(Suppl 2), II76–80.

Domschke, K., Zavorotnyy, M., Diemer, J. *et al.* (2010) COMT val158met influence on electroconvulsive therapy response in major depression. *Am. J. Med. Genet. B. Neuropsychiatr. Genet.*, **153B**(1), 286–290.

Drago, A., Crisafulli, C., Sidoti, A. *et al.* (2011) The molecular interaction between the glutamatergic, noradrenergic, dopaminergic and serotoninergic systems informs a detailed genetic perspective on depressive phenotypes. *Prog. Neurobiol.*, **94**(4), 418–460.

Dwivedi, Y., Rao, J. S., Rizavi, H. S. *et al.* (2003) Abnormal expression and functional characteristics of cyclic adenosine monophosphate response element binding protein in postmortem brain of suicide subjects. *Arch. Gen. Psychiatry*, **60**(3), 273–282.

Egan, M. F., Kojima, M., Callicott, J. H. *et al.* (2003) The BDNF val66met polymorphism affects activity-dependent secretion of BDNF and human memory and hippocampal function. *Cell*, **112**(2), 257–269.

Falkenberg, V. R., Gurbaxani, B. M., Unger, E. R. *et al.* (2011) Functional genomics of serotonin receptor 2A (HTR2A): interaction of polymorphism, methylation, expression and disease association. *Neuromolec. Med.*, **13**(1), 66–76.

Garriock, H. A., Allen, J. J., Delgado, P. *et al.* (2005) Lack of association of TPH2 exon XI polymorphisms with major depression and treatment resistance. *Mol. Psychiatry*, **10**(11), 976–977.

Gold, S. J., Heifets, B. D., Pudiak, C. M. *et al.* (2002) Regulation of regulators of G protein signaling mRNA expression in rat brain by acute and chronic electroconvulsive seizures. *J. Neurochem.*, **82**(4), 828–838.

Heurteaux, C., Lucas, G., Guy, N. *et al.* (2006) Deletion of the background potassium channel TREK-1 results in a depression-resistant phenotype. *Nat. Neurosci.*, **9**(9), 1134–1141.

Huuhka, M., Anttila, S., Leinonen, E. *et al.* (2005) The apolipoprotein E polymorphism is not associated with response to electroconvulsive therapy in major depressive disorder. *J. ECT*, **21**(1), 7–11.

Huuhka, K., Anttila, S., Huuhka, M. *et al.* (2007) Brain-derived neurotrophic factor (BDNF) polymorphisms G196A and C270T are not associated with response to electroconvulsive therapy in major depressive disorder. *Eur. Arch. Psychiatry Clin. Neurosci.*, **257**(1), 31–35.

Huuhka, K., Anttila, S., Huuhka, M. *et al.* (2008a) Dopamine 2 receptor C957T and catechol-o-methyltransferase Val158Met polymorphisms are associated with treatment response in electroconvulsive therapy. *Neurosci. Lett.*, **448**(1), 79–83.

Huuhka, K., Kampman, O., Anttila, S. *et al.* (2008b) RGS4 polymorphism and response to electroconvulsive therapy in major depressive disorder. *Neurosci. Lett.*, **437**(1), 25–28.

Jacobs, B. L., van Praag, H. & Gage, F. H. (2000) Adult brain neurogenesis and psychiatry: a novel theory of depression. *Mol. Psychiatry*, **5**(3), 262–269.

Kato, M. & Serretti, A. (2010) Review and meta-analysis of antidepressant pharmacogenetic findings in major depressive disorder. *Mol. Psychiatry*, **15**(5), 473–500.

Kishida, I., Aklillu, E., Kawanishi, C. *et al.* (2007) Monoamine metabolites level in CSF is related to the 5-HTT gene polymorphism in treatment-resistant depression. *Neuropsychopharmacol.*, **32**(10), 2143–2151.

Kocabas, N. A., Antonijevic, I., Faghel, C. *et al.* (2011) Brain-derived neurotrophic factor gene polymorphisms: influence on treatment response phenotypes of major depressive disorder. *Int. Clin. Psychopharmacol.*, **26**(1), 1–10.

Kocabas, N. A., Faghel, C., Barreto, M. *et al.* (2010) The impact of catechol-O-methyltransferase SNPs and haplotypes on treatment response phenotypes in major depressive disorder: a case-control association study. *Int. Clin. Psychopharmacol.*, **25**(4), 218–227.

Kocabas, N. A., Antonijevic, I., Faghel, C. *et al.* (2011) Dysbindin gene (DTNBP1) in major depressive disorder (MDD) patients: lack of association with clinical phenotypes. *World J. Biol. Psychiatry*, **11**(8), 985–990.

Levin, G. M., Bowles, T. M., Ehret, M. J. *et al.* (2007) Assessment of human serotonin 1A receptor polymorphisms and SSRI responsiveness. *Mol. Diagn. Ther.*, **11**(3), 155–160.

Lin, P. I., Vance, J. M., Pericak-Vance, M. A. *et al.* (2007) No gene is an island: the flip-flop phenomenon. *Am. J. Hum. Gen.*, **80**(3), 531–538.

Maier, W. & Zobel, A. (2008) Contribution of allelic variations to the phenotype of response to antidepressants and antipsychotics. *Eur. Arch. Psychiatry Clin. Neurosci.*, **258**(Suppl. 1), 12–20.

Malaguti, A., Rossini, D., Lucca, A. *et al.* (2011) Role of COMT, 5-HT(1A), and SERT genetic polymorphisms on antidepressant response to Transcranial Magnetic Stimulation. *Depression & Anxiety*, **28**(7), 568–573.

Mamdani, F., Lopez, J., Berlim, M. *et al.* (2011) *Transcriptomic and epigenetic correlates of antidepressant response*. XIXth World Congress of Psychiatric Genetics: Genes to Biology, Washington, DC, USA.

Mandelli, L., Mazza, M., Martinotti, G. *et al.* (2010) Further evidence supporting the influence of brain-derived neurotrophic factor on the outcome of bipolar depression: independent effect of brain-derived neurotrophic factor and harm avoidance. *J. Psychopharmacol.*, **24**(12), 1747–1754.

Manji, H. K., Quiroz, J. A., Sporn, J. *et al.* (2003) Enhancing neuronal plasticity and cellular resilience to develop novel, improved therapeutics for difficult-to-treat depression. *Biol. Psychiatry*, **53**(8), 707–742.

Minelli, A., Zanardini, R., Abate, M. *et al.* (2011) Vascular Endothelial Growth Factor (VEGF) serum concentration during electroconvulsive therapy (ECT) in treatment resistant depressed patients. *Prog. Neuropsychopharmacol. Biol. Psychiatry*, **35**(5), 1322–1325.

Noro, M., Antonijevic, I., Forray, C. *et al.* (2010) 5HT1A and 5HT2A receptor genes in treatment response phenotypes in major depressive disorder. *Int. Clin. Psychopharmacol.*, **25**(4), 228–231.

O'Brien, F. E., Dinan, T. G., Griffin, B. T. *et al.* (2011) Interactions between antidepressants and P-glycoprotein at the blood-brain barrier: clinical significance of in vitro and in vivo findings. *Brit. J. Pharmacol.*, doi:10.1111/j.1476-5381.2011.01557.x.

Paik, S., Tang, G., Shak, S. *et al.* (2006) Gene expression and benefit of chemotherapy in women with node-negative, estrogen receptor-positive breast cancer. *J. Clin. Oncol.*, **24**(23), 3726–3734.

Perlis, R. H., Moorjani, P., Fagerness, J. *et al.* (2008) Pharmacogenetic analysis of genes implicated in rodent models of antidepressant response: association of TREK1 and treatment resistance in the STAR(*)D study. *Neuropsychopharmacol.*, **33**(12), 2810–2819.

Porcelli, S., Drago, A., Fabbri, C. *et al.* (2011a) Mechanisms of antidepressant action: an integrated dopaminergic perspective. *Prog. Neuropsychopharmacol. Biol. Psychiatry*, **35**(7), 1532–1543.

Porcelli, S., Drago, A., Fabbri, C. *et al.* (2011b) Pharmacogenetics of antidepressant response. *J. Psychiatry Neurosci.*, **36**(2), 87–113.

Porcelli, S., Fabbri, C., Drago, A. *et al.* (2011c) Genetics and antidepressants: where we are. *Clin. Neuropsych.*, **8**(2), 99–150.

Porcelli, S., Fabbri, C., Spina, E. *et al.* (2011d) Genetic polymorphisms of cytochrome P450 enzymes and antidepressant metabolism. *Exp. Op. Drug Metab. Toxicol.*, **7**(9), 1101–1115.

Psychiatric GWAS Consortium Steering Committee (2009) A framework for interpreting genome-wide association studies of psychiatric disorders. *Mol. Psychiatry*, **14**(1), 10–17.

Reimherr, F., Amsterdam, J., Dunner, D. *et al.* (2010) Genetic polymorphisms in the treatment of depression: speculations from an augmentation study using atomoxetine. *Psy. Res.*, **175**(1–2), 67–73.

Richardson-Jones, J. W., Craige, C. P., Guiard, B. P. *et al.* (2010) 5-HT1A autoreceptor levels determine vulnerability to stress and response to antidepressants. *Neuron*, **65**(1), 40–52.

Roberts, R., Wells, G. A., Stewart, A. F. *et al.* (2010) The genome-wide association study – a new era for common polygenic disorders. *J. Cardio. Trans. Res.*, **3**(3), 173–182.

Rosenhagen, M. C. & Uhr, M. (2010) Single nucleotide polymorphism in the drug transporter gene ABCB1 in treatment-resistant depression: clinical practice. *J. Clin. Psychopharmacol.*, **30**(2), 209–211.

Sapolsky, R. M. (2000) The possibility of neurotoxicity in the hippocampus in major depression: a primer on neuron death. *Biol. Psychiatry*, **48**(8), 755–765.

Scharinger, C., Rabl, U., Pezawas, L. *et al.* (2011) The genetic blueprint of major depressive disorder: contributions of imaging genetics studies. *World J. Biol. Psychiatry*, **2**, 474–488.

Schosser, A., Calati, R., Serretti, A. *et al.* (2011) The impact of COMT gene polymorphisms on suicidality in treatment resistant major depressive disorder – a European Multicenter Study. *Eur. Neuropsychopharmacol*, **25**(4), 218–227.

Segi-Nishida, E. (2011) Exploration of new molecular mechanisms for antidepressant actions of electroconvulsive seizure. *Biol. Pharmaceut. Bull.*, **34**(7), 939–944.

Serretti, A., Franchini, L., Gasperini, M. *et al.* (1998) Mode of inheritance in mood disorders families according to fluvoxamine response. *Acta Psychiatr. Scand.*, **98**(6), 443–450.

Serretti, A., Kato, M. & Kennedy, J. L. (2008) Pharmacogenetic studies in depression: a proposal for methodologic guidelines. *Pharmacogen. J.*, **8**(2), 90–100.

Serretti, A., Chiesa, A., Calati, R. *et al.* (2011a) A preliminary investigation of the influence of CREB1 gene on treatment resistance in major depression. *J. Affect. Disord.*, **128**(1–2), 56–63.

Serretti, A., Chiesa, A., Calati, R. *et al.* (2011b) No influence of PTGS2 polymorphisms on response and remission to antidepressants in major depression. *Psy. Res.*, **188**(1), 166–169.

Serretti, A., Olgiati, P., Bajo, E. *et al.* (2011c) A model to incorporate genetic testing (5-HTTLPR) in pharmacological treatment of major depressive disorders. *World J. Biol. Psychiatry*, **12**(7), 501–515.

Shih, J. C., Chen, K. & Ridd, M. J. (1999) Role of MAO A and B in neurotransmitter metabolism and behavior. *Polish J. Pharmacol.*, **51**(1), 25–29.

Slodkowska, E. A. & Ross, J. S. (2009) MammaPrint 70-gene signature: another milestone in personalized medical care for breast cancer patients. *Exp. Rev. Mol. Diagnost.*, **9**(5), 417–422.

Steffensen, K. D., Waldstrom, M., Brandslund, I. *et al.* (2010) The relationship of VEGF polymorphisms with serum VEGF levels and progression-free survival in patients with epithelial ovarian cancer. *Gyn. Oncol.*, **117**(1), 109–116.

Stewart, J. A., Kampman, O., Huuhka, M. *et al.* (2009) ACE polymorphism and response to electroconvulsive therapy in major depression. *Neurosci. Lett.*, **458**(3), 122–125.

Sullivan, P. F. (2007) Spurious genetic associations. *Biol. Psychiatry*, **61**(10), 1121–1126.

Sullivan, P. F., Neale, M. C. & Kendler, K. S. (2000) Genetic epidemiology of major depression: review and meta-analysis. *Am. J. Psychiatry*, **157**(10), 1552–1562.

Trivedi, M. H., Rush, A. J., Wisniewski, S. R. *et al.* (2006) Evaluation of outcomes with citalopram for depression using measurement-based care in STAR*D: implications for clinical practice. *Am. J. Psychiatry*, **163**(1), 28–40.

Tsuang, M. S. F. (1990) *The Genetics of Mood Disorders.* Johns Hopkins University Press, Baltimore, MD, USA.

Uhr, M., Tontsch, A., Namendorf, C. *et al.* (2008) Polymorphisms in the drug transporter gene ABCB1 predict antidepressant treatment response in depression. *Neuron*, **57**(2), 203–209.

Viikki, M., Anttila, S., Kampman, O. *et al.* (2010a) Vascular endothelial growth factor (VEGF) polymorphism is associated with treatment resistant depression. *Neurosci. Lett.*, **477**(3), 105–108.

Viikki, M., Kampman, O., Illi, A. *et al.* (2010b) TPH1 218A/C polymorphism is associated with major depressive disorder and its treatment response. *Neurosci. Lett.*, **468**(1), 80–84.

Viikki, M., Kampman, O., Anttila, S. *et al.* (2011a) P2RX7 polymorphisms Gln460Arg and His155Tyr are not associated with major depressive disorder or remission after SSRI or ECT. *Neurosci. Lett.*, **493**(3), 127–130.

Viikki, M., Huuhka, K., Leinonen, E. *et al.* (2011b) Interaction between two HTR2A polymorphisms and gender is associated with treatment response in MDD. *Neurosci. Lett.*, **501**(1), 20–24.

Warner-Schmidt, J. L. & Duman, R. S. (2008) VEGF as a potential target for therapeutic intervention in depression. *Curr. Opin. Pharmacol.*, **8**(1), 14–19.

Wellcome Trust Case Control Consortium (2007) Genome-wide association study of 14,000 cases of seven common diseases and 3,000 shared controls. *Nature*, **447**(7145), 661–678.

Wilkie, M. J., Smith, D., Reid, I. C. *et al*. (2007) A splice site polymorphism in the G-protein beta subunit influences antidepressant efficacy in depression. *Pharmacogen. Gen.*, **17**(3), 207–215.

Xu, B., Roos, J. L., Dexheimer, P. *et al*. (2011) Exome sequencing supports a de novo mutational paradigm for schizophrenia. *Nat. Gen.*, **43**(9), 864–868.

Yu, H. & Chen, Z. Y. (2011) The role of BDNF in depression on the basis of its location in the neural circuitry. *Acta Pharmacol. Sinica*, **32**(1), 3–11.

Zanardi, R., Magri, L., Rossini, D. *et al*. (2007) Role of serotonergic gene polymorphisms on response to transcranial magnetic stimulation in depression. *Eur. Neuropsychopharmacol.*, **17**(10), 651–657.

Zarate, C. Jr, Machado-Vieira, R., Henter, I. *et al*. (2010) Glutamatergic modulators: the future of treating mood disorders? *Harvard Rev. Psychiatry*, **18**(5), 293–303.

Zhang, X., Gainetdinov, R. R., Beaulieu, J. M. *et al*. (2005) Loss-of-function mutation in tryptophan hydroxylase-2 identified in unipolar major depression. *Neuron*, **45**(1), 11–16.

CHAPTER 4

Is There a Role for Switching Antidepressants in Treatment-resistant Depression?

Stuart Montgomery

*Imperial College of Science, Technology and Medicine,
University of London, London, UK*

Summary

The commonest strategy employed in treating depression that has not responded to an antidepressant is to raise the dose. This strategy is misguided: several careful, randomised, high-dose-versus-low-dose double-blind studies have failed to show an advantage to raising the dose (Licht and Quitzan, 2002; Schweitzer *et al.*, 2001; Wernicke *et al.*, 1989). Raising the dose has several disadvantages in that it delays recognition of early-state resistant depression and increases the incidence of discontinuation symptoms if the failed medication is stopped.

Treatment-resistant Depression, First Edition. Edited by Siegfried Kasper and Stuart Montgomery.
© 2013 John Wiley & Sons, Ltd. Published 2013 by John Wiley & Sons, Ltd.

The second commonest strategy used in nonresponse is to switch to a different class of antidepressant. Again, several metaanalyses (Bschor & Baethge, 2010; Ruhe *et al.*, 2006; Rush *et al.*, 2006) have found that this practice confers no advantage. In a recent prospective study by Sourey *et al.* (2011), switching class showed a significant disadvantage. In the light of these results, we should update our practice, rewrite our guidelines and consider alternative strategies for treating resistant depression, such as using a superior antidepressant independent of class or using an augmentation strategy.

Introduction

When a physician is faced with a patient suffering from major depression who fails to respond to treatment with the prescribed antidepressant, the dilemma of what action to take must be addressed. Once issues such as compliance with treatment, tolerability and the possible influence of comorbid conditions have been investigated and ruled out, there appears to be a reliance on clinical habit, with a choice of either raising the dose of the antidepressant to increase its pharmacological action or switching treatment to an antidepressant of a different pharmacological class. The evidence to support either strategy is remarkably slender.

Raising the dose

Despite the frequent clinical practice of raising the dose of an antidepressant in nonresponding patients, identification of an improved chance of response has proved elusive. Dose-finding studies carried out with selective serotonin reuptake inhibitors (SSRIs) are consistent in showing that these antidepressants have a flat dose–response relationship, with no extra response observed at higher doses. Escitalopram may be an exception, since with this drug some improvement at higher doses has been reported (Gorman *et al.*, 2002). The issue has been investigated in careful randomized studies, carried out under double-blind conditions, in which the dose of antidepressant was raised in nonresponders versus not being raised. These studies have failed to find any improved efficacy on raising the dose (Dornseif *et al.*, 1989; Schweizer *et al.*, 2001; Wernicke *et al.*, 1989), and in one very large study the responder rate was reported to be significantly reduced (Licht & Qvitzau, 2002). A randomized open study on paroxetine also found no extra efficacy or benefit from raising the dose in nonresponders (Ruhe *et al.*, 2009).

Increasing the dose carries the inevitable risk of increasing the burden of adverse events, which have been shown to be dose-related. All studies have reported an increase in adverse events when the dose is raised, so that the benefit–risk ratio was negative: an increased risk of adverse events but no benefit in efficacy. It appears that all that is achieved by raising the dose is an increase in the risk of unwanted effects. A further disadvantage of increasing the dose is the likelihood of an increase in discontinuation symptoms when that treatment is eventually terminated, since these too are dose-related. Increasing the dose of antidepressant generally appears to be counterproductive for all patients, with the possible exception of the individual who is a fast metabolizer and who may therefore need the higher dose in order to achieve sufficient plasma levels of the antidepressant for it to be effective.

Switching antidepressant pharmacological class

At first sight, it may appear logical to change the antidepressant of a nonresponding depressed patient to one of a different pharmacological class. This strategy is based on the assumption that if an individual fails to respond to one pharmacological action, for example serotonin reuptake inhibition, they might respond to a different one. However, evidence from studies of currently available antidepressants in support of changing pharmacological class is weak. The concept that all members of a pharmacological class of antidepressants have similar actions is itself fallacious, and disregards the many studies that have demonstrated differences in action and in efficacy among antidepressants belonging to a particular pharmacological class. The concept also overlooks the heterogeneity of action of antidepressants from different classes despite the 'selective' terminology.

Serotonin norepinephrine reuptake inhibitors

The different members of the group of antidepressants labelled as 'serotonin norepinephrine reuptake inhibitors' (SNRIs) vary widely in their levels of reuptake inhibition of noradrenaline and serotonin. The level of noradrenaline reuptake inhibition ranges from trivial to equal to the level of inhibition of serotonin reuptake. An individual antidepressant is considered to be a member of the class of serotonin noradrenaline reuptake inhibitors provided it inhibits reuptake of both noradrenaline and serotonin, however minor the contribution of either may be. The oldest member of the SNRI class is venlafaxine, in which the ratio of serotonin reuptake to noradrenaline reuptake is reported to be 30 to 1 (Koch *et al.*, 2003). At the doses of venlafaxine customarily prescribed (for example, 75 and 150 mg), the amount of noradrenaline reuptake is so minimal that venlafaxine is considered to be in effect an SSRI (Blier *et al.*, 2007). The same applies to venlafaxine's active metabolite, desvenlafaxine, which accounts for the majority of the effects of venlafaxine and is also marketed as an SNRI. The dose recommended in the USA for desvenlafaxine is 50–100 mg a day, and at this level the amount of noradrenaline reuptake inhibition is likewise slight. In practice, it is probably incorrect to identify either venlafaxine or desvenlafaxine as an SNRI since at their most commonly used doses their actions are to all intents and purposes those of SSRIs.

Duloxetine, the third member of this class of SNRI, has slightly higher levels of noradrenaline reuptake inhibition than venlafaxine, but the ratio *in vitro* is still reported to be only 14 parts serotonin to one part noradrenaline (Koch *et al.*, 2003). The noradrenaline reuptake inhibition produced with the recommended dose of 60 mg of duloxetine is so minor that this antidepressant becomes an SNRI only at higher than the recommended doses. However, there is no evidence that these higher doses, for example 120 mg or above, have any advantage in efficacy over the lower dose of 60 mg (Brecht *et al.*, 2011), and in the EU, according to the formal assessment of the European Medicines Agency (EMA), duloxetine 60 mg is the only recommended dose.

The only true SNRI licensed in Europe is milnacipran, which has an approximately equal effect on both noradrenaline and serotonin receptors. This antidepressant is available only in a very limited number of countries in Europe and is not licensed as an antidepressant in the USA. Its S-enantiomer, levomilnacipran, is in late phase 3 development in the USA and, based on two positive studies showing a significant difference from placebo, is clearly an effective antidepressant. Levomilnacipran has marked effects on the core symptoms of depression, such as anhedonia and lack of energy, to which the efficacy of conventional SSRI antidepressants such as fluoxetine and paroxetine appears to be compromised (Montgomery *et al.*, 2010). This suggests that the extra efficacy against these symptoms is due to noradrenaline reuptake inhibition. These very promising data from the USA suggest that levomilnacipran will be an important member of the class of SNRIs, although given the apparent restrictions on licensing enantiomers in the EU, clinicians in Europe may not have the choice of prescribing this antidepressant.

Selective serotonin reuptake inhibitors

The idea that SSRIs are members of a distinct homogenous class of antidepressants with similar efficacies is even more difficult to sustain. In common with all members of the so-called

SNRI class of antidepressants, these compounds all have serotonin reuptake-inhibiting properties. However, evidence is accumulating that pharmacological activity and efficacy differ between compounds within this class. Recommendations for treatment based on class of antidepressant alone may therefore be unhelpful, since the evidence that some SSRIs have well-documented superior efficacy compared to others may be overlooked.

In this group, escitalopram is unique in its effect of binding to the allosteric binding site on the serotonin transporter, which stabilizes and increases binding on the primary reuptake site. From a series of elegant studies on the pharmacology of citalo-pram, it is clear that the inactive R-enantiomer present in this antidepressant blocks the binding of the S-enantiomer to the serotonin transporter, disabling the allosteric mechanism (Sanchez, 2006). It is for this reason that the S-enantiomer esci-talopram is a different and more effective antidepressant than the racemate citalopram, with its mixture of R and S enantiom-ers. Escitalopram has been shown to be more effective than equivalent doses of citalopram at a clinically relevant level in two ground-breaking studies (Moore et al., 2005; Yevtushenko et al., 2007). Escitalopram has also been shown to be more effective than paroxetine in both the short term (12 weeks) and the long term (6 months) (Boulenger et al., 2006). Greater effi-cacy and better tolerability compared to the so-called SNRI duloxetine (Khan et al., 2007; Lam et al., 2008; Wade et al., 2007), and compared to venlafaxine in severe depression (Montgomery & Andersen, 2006), are reported for escitalo-pram. The superiority of escitalopram in these studies passed stringent criteria for clinical relevance (Montgomery & Moller, 2009). The simplistic concept that all SSRIs are the same is not sustainable when the results of these studies are taken into account. The data suggest that rather than switching treatment of a nonresponding patient to an antidepressant of a different pharmacological class, a better strategy might be to switch from a conventional SSRI to escitalopram, as suggested by Lam et al. (2010) and reviewed by Montgomery & Möller (2009).

Other SSRIs also differ in their pharmacological activity; for example, sertraline has substantial dopamine effects and both sertraline and fluvoxamine have sigma-antagonistic activity. Fluoxetine is a 5-HT$_{2C}$ receptor agonist, which is thought to explain why it appears to provoke substantial anxiety, an effect that has compromised its efficacy in generalized anxiety disorder (GAD). Paroxetine has the most marked sedative effect of all the SSRIs, due probably to its activity on H$_1$ antagonism.

These clear differences in pharmacological action limit the perception of the so-called SSRIs as a distinct and homogenous class of antidepressants, each with the same level of efficacy, and call into question the assumption of parity which appears to underlie guidelines such as those of the UK National Institute for Health and Clinical Excellence (NICE) (http://www.nice.org.uk/Guidance/CG23). There is now a substantial body of evidence on the efficacy of different antidepressants, sufficient to discourage prescription by pharmacological class and to suggest focusing instead on tailoring treatment to the individual patient, taking into account the evidence that some individual antidepressants are better than others.

Guidelines on second-step treatment of nonresponders

Numerous guidelines make recommendations as to which antidepressants should be used as first-line treatment and which should be considered as a second or even third step. Very few are based on a considered analysis of the data reported from recent studies. In general, current guidelines for the treatment of nonresponding depression make recommendations that are based on grouping antidepressants into pharmacological classes. This guidance does not analyse the available studies to determine whether the concept of a pharmacological class of antidepressant is useful in the management of nonresponse or treatment-resistant depression (TRD).

It is understandable in the present economic climate, though regrettable, that some of the guidelines published appear to be more concerned with the costs of antidepressants than with the scientific data showing differences in efficacy between them. The expertise of prescribers is not reflected in the guidance so much as decisions emanating from government or health-insurance bodies, which, in order to restrict costs, recommend only generic SSRIs. The burden of depression and the high costs of nonresponse for the individual, the family and society at large are generally not discussed or taken into account. An obvious example is the guidelines issued by NICE: input from a body of prescribers is not sought and there is a general absence of specialist expertise. For example, there was no psychiatrist member of the large committee to produce the NICE guidelines on the use of electroconvulsive therapy (ECT) in psychiatry. This failure to have an adequate input from experts renders the guidance unsafe and unreliable. A similar criticism can be levelled at other bodies that have rationing by cost as their primary goal, for example the compulsory prescription guidelines in Germany or the Transparency Commission on Reimbursement in France and other countries.

A series of independent guidelines on TRD that have been produced by specialists, for example the definitions of Thase & Rush (1997), the Massachusetts General Hospital staging model (MGH-S) (Fava, 2003), the British Association of Psychopharmacology guidelines (Anderson *et al.*, 2008) and the World Federation of Societies of Biological Psychiatry guidelines (Bauer *et al.*, 2002), all make the assumption that prescribing by pharmacological class is acceptable and that switching class is recommended for nonresponse. The only exception is published by the Group for the Study of Resistant Depression (GSRD) (Souery *et al.*, 1999), which defines TRD by the number of periods of treatment with any antidepressant, regardless of pharmacological class, and not by whether there has been a switch of the class of antidepressant prescribed. There is obviously a need for evidence-based guidance that examines the scientific literature and makes recommendations from the evidence base.

Does switching class of antidepressant improve response?

A number of studies have investigated this issue but the results have not yet been incorporated into any formal guidance. A metaanalysis comparing the benefit of switching to a different pharmacological class with the benefit of switching to an antidepressant within the same class concluded that switching class showed no advantage (Ruhe *et al.*, 2006). Similar results were reported in an analysis of three studies, in which staying on the same antidepressant had comparable efficacy to switching to a different class (Bschor & Baethge, 2010). In the very large Sequenced Treatment Alternatives to Relieve Depression (STAR*D) study, in which the choice of second treatment was left to practitioners and patients, there was no evidence that switching class of antidepressant was beneficial (Rush *et al.*, 2006). Analysis of the large dataset of the GSRD found that switching the class of antidepressant was associated with a worse outcome – although the difference did not reach significance – than switching antidepressants within the same class; the responder rate in the group treated within antidepressant class was 47.5%, compared with 40% in the group switching to a different class (Souery *et al.*, 2011a). A prospective test of second-step treatment reported that in those who failed the first antidepressant (almost entirely SSRIs), switching to escitalopram was associated with a significantly better responder and remission rate than switching to the SNRIs venlafaxine or duloxetine, with a fourfold lower responder rate seen on the SNRIs (Lam *et al.*, 2010).

Only one report has found the opposite effect, in a retrospective metaanalysis of four studies which individually were not significant (Papakostas *et al.*, 2008). In this analysis, remission was significantly more likely in the group that switched class of

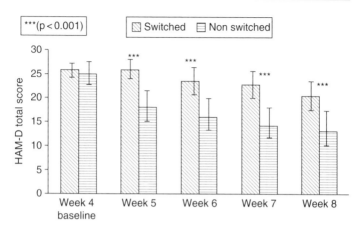

Figure 4.1   Treatment-resistant depression (TRD) patients randomized to treatment for 4 weeks with citalopram or desipramine. Nonresponders at 4 weeks were randomized to switch to alternative treatment or remain on the same treatment. Data from Souery *et al.* (2011b)

antidepressant. However, this study failed to find a difference in the more usual responder analysis.

The GSRD has recently published the results of a prospective study investigating the effects of switching antidepressant in TRD (Souery *et al.*, 2011b). This was a very focused study, in that it explored the effect not just of switching class of antidepressant but also of switching to a different mechanism, since patients were switched from treatment with desipramine, a TCA with noradrenaline reuptake-inhibition properties, to the SSRI citalopram, or vice versa. Patients with TRD who failed to respond to each antidepressant were randomly switched to the opposite class or kept on the same class, persisting with the same treatment.

The results showed that in TRD, switching class and mechanism after 4 weeks' treatment was associated with significantly poorer response than staying on the same antidepressant for a further 4 weeks (Figure 4.1). In order to answer the potential criticism that the doses used were too low, the dose of antidepressant was increased: 200 mg for desipramine and 40–60 mg for citalopram. In retrospect, this might have been a mistake, since the abrupt switch appeared to be associated with withdrawal effects for both antidepressants, which may have interfered with subsequent response. Nevertheless, the results of this prospective study show that the strategy of switching antidepressants to a different class in at 4 weeks nonresponders is associated with a significantly poorer subsequent outcome than remaining on the same treatment. Switching the class and mechanism of action in TRD in this study produced the poorer outcome (Figure 4.1).

The overall evidence from these different studies, which used different methodologies in varying populations, is that switching the class of antidepressant does not produce a better outcome than remaining on the same class. In almost all studies there was no advantage (Bschor & Baethge, 2010; Ruhe *et al.*, 2006; Souery *et al.*, 2011a) and in the only prospective study there was a significant disadvantage in switching class, measured by both response and remission (Souery *et al.*, 2011b). In one study there was a small advantage to switching seen in remission alone, but not in response (Papakostas *et al.*, 2008). The overall evidence does not support the widely recommended advice to switch the class of antidepressant in the case of nonresponse or treatment resistance to antidepressants.

These data were reviewed in an EMA concept paper (Broich, 2009). Both the concept paper and the recently released EMA draft guidelines for the treatment of depression omit the advice of previous guidelines that the definition of treatment resistance in the EU for patients entering studies on the treatment of TRD should include failure to respond to a switch in the class of antidepressant.

Conclusions

It is time to investigate alternative strategies for the second-step treatment of nonresponders to antidepressants and to produce new advice on the definition and treatment of TRD. Treating

TRD by the class of antidepressant and its presumed mechanism of action clearly does not optimize response and may even worsen it. Whether this is due to reactions associated with the withdrawal of the previous antidepressant, to a very slow response to the new antidepressant or to some other mechanism is not clear. It is however clear that switching the class of antidepressant in nonresponders or in TRD is not supported by the data.

References

Anderson, I. M., Ferrier, I. N., Baldwin, R. C. *et al*. (2008) Evidence-based guidelines for treating depressive disorders with antidepressants: a revision of the 2000 British Association for Psychopharmacology guidelines. *J. Psychopharmacol.*, **22**, 343–396.

Bauer, M., Whybrow, P. C., Angst, J. *et al*. (2002) World Federation of Societies of Biological Psychiatry (WFSBP) Gguidelines for biological treatment of unipolar depressive disorders, Part 1: Acute and continuation treatment of major depressive disorder. *World J. Biol. Psychiatry*, **3**, 5–43.

Blier, P., Saint-André, E., Hébert, C. *et al*. (2007) Effects of different doses of venlafaxine on serotonin and norepinephrine reuptake in healthy volunteers. *Int. J. Neuropsychopharmacol.*, **10**, 41–50.

Boulenger, J.-P., Huusom, A. K. T., Florea, I. *et al*. (2006) A comparative study of the efficacy of long-term treatment with escitalopram and paroxetine in severely depressed patients. *Curr. Med. Res. Opin.*, **22**, 1331–1341.

Brecht, S., Desaiah, D., Marechal, E. S. *et al*. (2011) Efficacy and safety of duloxetine 60 mg and 120 mg daily in patients hospitalized for severe depression: a double-blind randomized trial. *J. Clin. Psychiatry*, **72**, 1086–1094.

Broich, K. (2009) Committee for Medicinal Products for Human Use (CHMP) assessment of efficacy of antidepressants. *Eur. Neuropsychopharmacol.*, **19**, 305–308.

Bschor, T. & Baethge, C. (2010) No evidence for switching the antidepressant:systematic review and meta-analysis of RCTs of a common therapeutic strategy. *Acta Psychiatr. Scand.*, **121**, 174–179.

Dornseif, B. E., Dunlop, S. R., Potvin, J. H. & Wernicke, J. F. (1989) Effect of dose escalation after low-dose fluoxetine therapy. *Psychopharmacol. Bull.*, **25**, 71–79.

Fava, M. (2003) Diagnosis and definition of treatment-resistant depression. *Biol. Psychiatry*, **53**, 649–659.

Gorman, J. M., Korotzer, A. & Su, G. (2002) Efficacy comparison of escitalopram and citalopram in the treatment of major depressive disorder: pooled analysis of placebo-controlled trials. *CNS Spectrum*, **7**, 40–44.

Khan, A., Bose, A., Alexopoulos, G. S. *et al.* (2007) Double-blind comparison of escitalopram and duloxetine in the acute treatment of major depressive disorder. *Clin. Drug Inves.*, **27**, 481–492.

Koch, S., Hemrick-Luecke, S. K., Thompson, L. K. *et al.* (2003) Comparison of effects of dual transporter inhibitors on monoamine transporters and extracellular levels in rats. *Neuropharmacol.*, **45**, 935–944.

Lam, R. W., Andersen, H. F. & Wade, A. G. (2008) Escitalopram and duloxetine in the treatment of major depressive disorder: a pooled analysis of two trials. *Int. Clin. Psychopharmacol.*, **23**, 181–187.

Lam, R. W., Lönn, S. L. & Despiegel, N. (2010) Escitalopram versus noradrenaline reuptake inhibitors as second step treatment for patients with major depressive disorder: a pooled analysis. *Int. Clin. Psychopharmacol.*, **25**, 199–203.

Licht, R. W. & Qvitzau, S. (2002) Treatment strategies in patients with major depression not responding to first-line sertraline treatment. A randomised study of extended duration of treatment, dose increase or mianserin augmentation. *Psychopharmacol. (Berlin)*, **161**, 143–151.

Montgomery, S., Lecrubier, Y., Mansuy, L. *et al.* (2010) Efficacy of levomilnacipran in improving symptoms and functional impairment associated with major depressive disorder. 163rd APA Meeting, New Orleans, LA, USA.

Montgomery, S. A. & Andersen, H. F. (2006) Escitalopram versus venlafaxine XR in the treatment of depression. *Int. Clin. Psychopharmacol.*, **21**, 297–309.

Montgomery, S. A. & Moller, H. J. (2009) Is the significant superiority of escitalopram compared with other antidepressants clinically relevant? *Int. Clin. Psychopharmacol.*, **24**, 111–118.

Moore, N., Verdoux, H. & Fantino, B. (2005) Prospective, multicentre, randomized, double-blind study of the efficacy of escitalopram versus citalopram in outpatient treatment of major depressive disorder. *Int. Clin. Psychopharmacol.*, **20**, 131–137.

Papakostas, G. I., Fava, M. & Thase, M. E. (2008) Treatment of SSRI-resistant depression: a meta-analysis comparing within- versus across-class switches. *Biol. Psychiatry*, **63**, 699–704.

Ruhe, H. G., Booij, J., van Weert, H. C. *et al.* (2009) Evidence why paroxetine dose escalation is not effective in major depressive disorder: a randomised controlled trial with assessment of serotonin transporter occupancy. *Neuropsychopharmacol.*, **34**, 999–1010.

Ruhe, H. G., Huyser, J., Swinkels, J. A., *et al.* (2006) Switching antidepressants after a first selective serotonin reuptake inhibitor in major depressive disorder: a systematic review. *J. Clin. Psychiatry*, **67**, 1836–1855.

Rush, A. J., Trivedi, M., Wisniewski, S. R. *et al.* (2006) Acute and longer-term outcomes in depressed outpatients requiring one or several treatment steps: a STAR*D report. *Am. J. Psychiatry*, **163**, 1905–1917.

Sanchez, C. (2006) The pharmacology of citalopram enantiomers: the antagonism of R-citalopram on the effect of S-citalopram. *Basic Clin. Toxicol.*, **99**, 91–95.

Schweizer, E., Rynn, M., Mandos, L. *et al.* (2001) The antidepressant effect of sertraline is not enhanced by dose titration: results from an outpatient clinical trial. *Int. Clin. Psychopharmacol.*, **16**, 137–143.

Souery, D., Amsterdam, J. D., Montigny, C. *et al.* (1999) Treatment resistant depression: methodological overview and operational criteria. *Eur. Neuropsychopharmacol.*, **9**, 83–91.

Souery, D., Serretti, A., Calati, R. *et al.* (2011a) Switching antidepressant class does not improve response or remission in treatment-resistant depression. *J. Clin. Psychopharmacol.*, **31**, 512–516.

Souery, D., Serretti, A., Calati, R. *et al.* (2011b) Citalopram versus desipramine in treatment resistant depression: effect of continuation or switching strategies: a randomized open study. *World J. Biol. Psychiatry*, **12**, 364–375.

Thase, M. E. & Rush, A. J. (1997) When at first you don't succeed: sequential strategies for antidepressant nonresponders. *J. Clin. Psychiatry Suppl.*, **13**, 23–29.

Wade, A. G., Gembert, K. & Florea, I. (2007) A comparative study of the efficacy of acute and continuation treatment with escitalopram versus duloxetine in patients with major depressive disorder. *Curr. Med. Res. Op.*, **23**, 1605–1614.

Wernicke, J. F., Bosomworth, J. C. & Ashbrook, E. (1989) Fluoxetine at 20 mg per day. I. The recommended and therapeutic dose in the treatment of depression. *Int. Clin. Psychopharmacol.*, **4**(Suppl. 1), 63–68.

Yevtushenko, V., Belous, A. I., Yevtushenko, Y. G. *et al.* (2007) Efficacy and tolerability of escitalopram versus citalopram in major depressive disorder: a 6-week, multicenter, prospective, randomized, double-blind, active-controlled study in adult outpatients. *Clin. Therapeutic.*, **29**, 19–32.

CHAPTER 5

The Role of Atypical Antipsychotics in Inadequate-response and Treatment-resistant Depression

Siegfried Kasper and Elena Akimova

*Department of Psychiatry and Psychotherapy,
Medical University of Vienna, Vienna, Austria*

Summary

Atypical antipsychotics, or second-generation antipsychotics (SGAs) as they are also called, have been introduced for the treatment of schizophrenia and, subsequently, for bipolar disorder. Although no formal indication exists, clinicians have begun to use them for the treatment of depression, as demonstrated in a large drug surveillance programme of German-speaking countries from 1997 onwards, which revealed that 43–46% of nonpsychotic depressed inpatients received SGAs and neuroleptics in addition to antidepressant medication.

Treatment-resistant Depression, First Edition. Edited by Siegfried Kasper and Stuart Montgomery.
© 2013 John Wiley & Sons, Ltd. Published 2013 by John Wiley & Sons, Ltd.

Substantial research on the combination therapy of antidepressants and SGAs has revealed that they are a valuable addition to antidepressant therapy. As a result of these studies, quetiapine has been approved in Europe as an add-on medication to ongoing antidepressant treatment in patients with a suboptimal response to antidepressants. In the USA, aripiprazole has also been granted indication for the adjunctive treatment of major depression, and olanzapin has the indication for combination with fluoxetine in treatment-resistant depression (TRD). Although a number of questions remain, it is apparent that the appropriate use of SGAs is a promising option for treatment in depression.

Introduction

Typical neuroleptics (TNs) and atypical antipsychotics, which are henceforth termed 'second-generation antipsychotics' (SGAs) in this chapter, have been used as an augmentation therapy for depression for a long time, starting with clozapine and haloperidol or low-potency neuroleptic agents (Bauer *et al.*, 2007; Chen *et al.*, 2011; Fava, 2001; Konstantinidis *et al.*, 2007; Philip *et al.*, 2010; Shelton & Papakostas, 2008). However, the recognition of extra-pyramidal side effects and the subsequent risk of tardive dyskinesia discouraged the continued use of TNs (Corell *et al.*, 2004; Goodwin *et al.*, 2009; Nelson, 1987).

With the introduction of SGAs and the experiences gained with clozapine, a new emphasis was placed on augmentation strategy with these agents as a treatment modality. The first systematic report on SGAs and augmentation therapy in major depressive disorder (MDD) was written by Ostroff & Nelson (1999), who described nonresponders to selective serotonin reuptake inhibitors (SSRIs) reacting rapidly when low doses of risperidone were supplemented. Thereafter, a placebo-controlled trial was conducted by Shelton *et al.* (2001), in which the combination of olanzapine and fluoxetine was demonstrated to be more effective than either drug alone in a sample of 30 patients resistant to treatment with fluoxetine alone. Since then, a number of studies have been undertaken in which different SGAs have been used as augmentation strategies, and as a result of this endeavour aripiprazole was the first SGA to be approved by the US Food and Drug Administration (FDA) for use as an augmentation agent in MDD, in the year 2008. Thereafter, olanzapine in combination with fluoxetine and quetiapine was given the same approval. In Europe, only quetiapine XR has been granted indication for inadequate response to treatment.

The different trials carried out so far with the SGAs olanzapine, risperidone, quetiapine and aripiprazole have used different definitions of prior failed trials, as outlined in Table 5.1. The definitions of 'two historical trials and one prospective trial', 'one or more historical trial and one prospective trial', 'one 4-week prospective trial', 'one historical trial of at least 3 weeks', 'one prospective trial of at least 5 weeks or a clearly documented trial', 'at least one historical trial of at least 6 weeks', 'one prior trial of at least 4 weeks and at least 6 weeks in the current trial', 'one or more trials of at least 6 weeks', 'one historical trial of at least six weeks' and 'one to three historical trials and one prospective trial' are examples of how these data have been obtained.

For practical as well as research reasons, it is therefore important to define the different treatment responses, as outlined in Table 5.2. Needless to say, the pathophysiology of depression is multifaceted and, as in other fields of medicine, requires different treatment modalities.

As indicated, an *inadequate response* would refer to an insufficient response to one therapy, usually lasting between 4 and 6 weeks. For this clinical characterization, quetiapine has been granted an indication by both the FDA and the European Medicines Agency (EMA). *Treatment nonresponse* would mean insufficient response to two therapies, ideally two prospective trials, although one historical and one prospective trial and two retrospective historical trials have been used in some studies. Most of the patients admitted to psychiatric inpatient treatment fulfil this criterion, and it is therefore obvious that depressed patients in psychiatric inpatient services have

Table 5.1 Augmentation trials with atypical antipsychotics (SGAs, second-generation antipsychotics) in treatment-resistant depression (TRD). Data included in a metaanalysis by Nelson & Papakostas (2009), reprinted with permission

Authors	Year	Atypical antipsychotic	Anti-depressant	N^a	Duration[b] (weeks)	Prior failed trials	Rating scale[c]
Shelton et al.	2001	Olanzapine	Fluoxetine	20	8	Two historical trials and one prospective trial	MADRS
Shelton et al.	2005	Olanzapine	Fluoxetine	288	8	One or more historical trial and one prospective trial	MADRS
Corya et al.	2006	Olanzapine	Fluoxetine	286	12	One or more historical trial and one prospective trial	MADRS
Thase et al.[d]	2007	Olanzapine	Fluoxetine	206	8	One or more historical trial and one prospective trial	MADRS
Thase et al.[d]	2007	Olanzapine	Fluoxetine	200	8	One or more historical trial and one prospective trial	MADRS
Mahmoud et al.	2007	Risperidone	Various	268	6	One 4-week prospective trial	HAM-D
Reeves et al.	2008	Risperidone	Various	23	8	One historical trial of at least 3 weeks	MADRS
Keitner et al.	2009	Risperidone	Various	95	4	One prospective trial of at least 5 weeks or a clearly documented trial	MADRS

Study	Year	Drug	Comparator	n[a]	Duration (weeks)[b]	Treatment history	Scale
Khullar et al.	2006	Quetiapine	SSRI/SNRI	15	8	At least one historical trial of at least 6 weeks	MADRS
Mattingly et al.	2006	Quetiapine	SSRI/SNRI	37	8	One prior trial of at least 4 weeks and at least 6 weeks in the current trial	MADRS
McIntyre et al.	2007	Quetiapine	SSRI/SNRI	58	8	One or more trials of at least 6 weeks	HAM-D
Earley et al.	2007	Quetiapine	SSRI/SNRI	487	6	One historical trial of at least 6 weeks	MADRS
El-Khalili et al.	2008	Quetiapine	SSRI/SNRI	432	8	One historical trial of at least 6 weeks	MADRS
Berman et al.	2007	Aripiprazole	SSRI/SNRI	353	6	One to three historical trials and one prospective trial	MADRS
Marcus et al.	2008	Aripiprazole	SSRI/SNRI	369	6	One to three historical trials and one prospective trial	MADRS
Berman et al.	2008	Aripiprazole	SSRI/SNRI	343	6	One to three historical trials and one prospective trial	MADRS

[a] Number of randomized patients with at least one post-treatment rating.

[b] Duration of the acute-phase double-blind controlled trial.

[c] HAM-D = Hamilton Depression Rating Scale; MADRS = Montgomery–Åsberg Depression Rating Scale.

[d] This report included two seperate trials of identical design.

Table 5.2   Definitions of treatment response

Treatment response	Definition
Inadequate response	Insufficient response to one therapy
Treatment nonresponse	Insufficient response to two therapies
Treatment refractory	Insufficient response to 'more' treatment options
Chronic depression	Depression over two years

received this treatment, as will be demonstrated later. *Treatment refractory depression* means insufficient response to 'more' treatment options – at least three treatment options, including electroconvulsive therapy (ECT) in some research papers. Studies performing deep-brain stimulation (DBS) used this criterion for the selection of their patients and included the additional requirement that these patients had failed to respond to ECT. Additionally, *chronic depression* needs to be characterized as a depression that lasts for more than 2 years. Interestingly, in the Sequenced Treatment Alternatives to Relieve Depression (STAR*D) study (Rush *et al.*, 2006), most of the patients fulfilled this criterion, since the mean length of duration of the indexed episode was more than 150 weeks.

From a pharmacological point of view, SGAs share some common properties, but also have distinctive differences (Farah, 2005; Kasper, 1998; Reynolds, 2004). All of them display a 5-HT2 receptor antagonism, but their relative potency varies. Additionally, aripiprazole and ziprasidone display a 5-HT1A partial antagonism (Stahl, 2003). All of the SGAs exhibit dopamine D2 receptor affinity and it is noteworthy that aripiprazole acts as a partial agonist at this receptor (Tadori *et al.*, 2008). With regard to the dopaminergic system, fast dissociation, as in the case of quetiapine, and preferential limbic D2 blockade, also not fully understood, play an important role. Further aminergic mechanisms such as noradrenalin and/or serotonin reuptake inhibition, as in the case of ziprasidone, zotepine and quetiapine, are vital in the treatment of these compounds in depression (Dunner *et al.*, 2007; El Khalili *et al.*, 2010). For instance, the metabolite of quetiapine, N-disalkyl quetiapine, has demonstrated an affinity for the norepinephrine reuptake transporter similar to that of duloxetine (Jensen *et al.*, 2008). Additionally, the combination of olanzapine and fluoxetine has demonstrated an increase in extracellular levels of dopamine and norepinephrine in animal experiments. This is important insofar as the agent alone or in combination with other SGAs and SSRIs did not demonstrate this effect (Zhang *et al.*, 2000). Ziprasidone has been associated with not only 5-HT1A partial agonism but also binding potential on the transporters dopamine, norepinephrine and serotonin in preclinical trials (Tatsumi *et al.*, 1999). These pharmacodynamic properties are thought to contribute to clinical efficacy. The effect of these compounds on α1 adrenergic, antihistaminergic and antimuscarinergic activity is associated with their side effects. In this chapter, the clinical evidence in everyday practice as well as the efficacy and side effects are described in more detail.

Epidemiology: prescription data

The available prescription data indicate that SGAs are used in depressed patients before official indication is obtained (Mohamed *et al.*, 2009). Philip *et al.* (2008) report that SGAs are used in depression, specifically for the treatment of agitation and insomnia. Olfson & Marcus (2009) and Lenderts & Kalali (2009) report an increase of SGAs in the USA between 1996 and 2005 and between 2008 and 2009, respectively. Two UK-based studies published in 2003 report a 16% increase in the use of SGAs from 1991 to 2000 (Kaye *et al.*, 2003) as well as widespread off-label use of SGAs in unipolar depression between 1997 and 1999 (Wheeler Vega *et al.*, 2003).

The largest amount of data so far available is the retrospective analysis based on the data obtained from the anonymized AMSP (Arzneimittelsicherheit in der Psychiatrie) International Pharmacovigilance databank, with reference-day data from all participating institutions in Austria, Germany and Switzerland. In this programme, the daily doses for psychotropic drugs are recorded on two reference days per hospital and per year, among other standardized variables (Grohmann *et al.*, 2004). In this dataset, the prescription patterns of 54 institutions were available in 2007, and of fewer than this in the years 2000 and 1997. The analysis included all depressed inpatients with one of the following diagnoses: ICD-10: F32.0, F32.00, F32.01, F32.1, F32.10, F32.11, F32.2, F33.0, F33.00, F33.01, F33.1, F33.10, F33.11 and F33.2. However, patients with psychotic subtypes were excluded from the analysis. In the article by Konstantinidis *et al.* (2012), the dataset from between 2000 and 2007 was published; the dataset from 1997 is also available as unpublished data. In Figure 5.1 it is apparent that 84–89% of the inpatients received antidepressant medication, and from 1997 onwards 43–46% of nonpsychotic depressed inpatients also received antipsychotic medication, which was either TNs or SGAs. Table 5.3 lists the most commonly used antipsy-chotics for depressed inpatients between 1997 and 2007. It is apparent that in 1997, haloperidol and promethazine were the most commonly prescribed agents, followed by olanzapine and promethazine in 2001, while in 2007 quetiapine, olanzapine and risperidone were the most prescribed. Furthermore, both high-potency and low-potency medication was used, mostly in dosages well below the schizophrenia and bipolar disorder indication. Olanzapine 8 mg, risperidone 2 mg and quetiapine 200 mg were the leading dosages.

According to the dataset available from AMSP, there was a significant increase in the prescription of SGAs in the total group as well as in the subgroup of inpatients with mild to mod-erate depression. This was astonishing insofar as the literature suggested there was only an indication for the addition of SGAs in severe depression. However, no data exist to date to show that patients suffering from mild to moderate depression also benefit from this treatment strategy. The database did not allow analysis of why these medications were used (for example, agitation or sleep problems), but it is very likely that clinicians

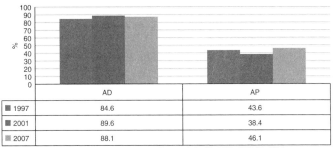

	AD	AP
■ 1997	84.6	43.6
■ 2001	89.6	38.4
■ 2007	88.1	46.1

Number of patients included in each group: 1997: N = 710; 2001: N = 1451; 2007: N = 2211
Diagnosis included: F32.*, F32.0, F32.00, F32.01, F32.1, F32.10, F32.11, F32.2, F32.8,
F32.9, F33.*, F33.0, F33.00, F33.01, F33.1, F33.10, F33.11, F33.2, F33.4, F33.8, F33.9

Figure 5.1   Use of antipsychotics (APs; typical as well as SGAs) and antidepressants (ADs) in depressive inpatients (1997–2007) in Germany, Austria and Switzerland. Data from Konstantinidis *et al.* (2012), reprinted with permission

Table 5.3   Most commonly used antipsychotics (Aps; typical as well as SGAs) in depressive inpatients (1997–2007) in Germany, Austria and Switzerland. Data from Konstantinidis *et al.* (2012), reprinted with permission

1997	2001	2007
Haloperidol 18.1% (6 mg)	Olanzapine 19.7% (8 mg)	Quetiapine 27.1% (232 mg)
Promethazine 13.9% (68 mg)	Promethazine 14.2% (80 mg)	Olanzapine 18.1% (10 mg)
Melperone 12.6% (75 mg)	Risperidone 13.6% (2 mg)	Promethazine 11.7% (66 mg)
Perozine 9.7% (198 mg)	Melperone 10.8% (62 mg)	Risperidone 10.2% (2 mg)
Chlorprothixen 7.7% (76 mg)	Pipamperone 8.5% (59 mg)	Pipamperone 10.1% (52 mg)

Number of patients included in each group: 1997 = 710; 2001 = 1451; 2007 = 2211
Diagnoses included: F32.*, F32.0, F32.00, F32.01, F32.1, F32.10, F32.11, F32.2, F32.8, F32.9, F33.*, F33.0, F33.00, F33.01, F33.1, F33.10, F33.11, F33.2, F33.4, F33.8, F33.9.
Terms in brackets show the mean dosage of antipsychotic per depressive inpatient, in mg.

were aware of the additional benefit of this medication and based their decision on experience as well as on its pharmaco-dynamic properties.

Efficacy of SGAs in TRD

The most thorough reviews and metaanalyses have been obtained by Papakostas *et al.* (2007) and Nelson & Papakostas (2009). Table 5.1 outlines the basic data of 16 studies used by the latter authors; the trials of ziprasidone, paliperidone, asenap-ine and iloperidone were not included, since they were not available at the time of publication. From the data available, the definition of how prior failed trials have been defined is of crucial importance. In more recent studies, such as those on quetiapine and aripiprazole, a more distinct characterization has been established. As already outlined, the distinction between inadequate response and treatment resistance should be made *a priori*, since different results are likely to be obtained with different definitions. Probably the best definition for treat-ment resistance is one historical trial and one prospective trial, not including agents that have been used before. If more than one historical trial or a definition of at least one historical trial is used, the likelihood that chronic depression is included and therefore that lower response rates are obtained is high.

In the metaanalysis conducted by Nelson & Papakostas (2009), response (e.g. reduction of MADRS total scores below 50% of baseline scores) and remission rates as defined in each individual trial (most likely MADRS total score below 11) were used as an outcome measure. Based on this definition, response and remis-sion rates for the total group showed a statistically significant advantage for the use of SGAs in addition to SSRIs and/or sero-tonin norepinephrine reuptake inhibitors (SNRIs) (see Figure 5.2).

Figure 5.3 gives an example of augmentation therapy with the SGA quetiapine when patients did not respond to a trial with SSRIs or SNRIs (McIntyre *et al.*, 2007). For this 8-week augmentation strategy the patient received either quetiapine

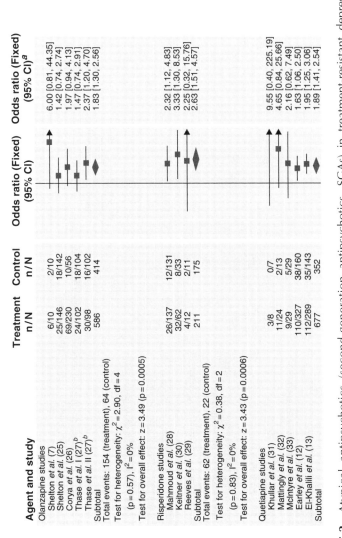

Agent and study	Treatment n/N	Control n/N	Odds ratio (Fixed) (95% CI)	Odds ratio (Fixed) (95% CI)[a]
Olanzapine studies				
Shelton et al. (7)	6/10	2/10		6.00 [0.81, 44.35]
Shelton et al. (25)	25/146	18/142		1.42 [0.74, 2.74]
Corya et al. (26)	69/230	10/56		1.97 [0.94, 4.13]
Thase et al. I (27)[b]	24/102	18/104		1.47 [0.74, 2.91]
Thase et al. II (27)[b]	30/98	16/102		2.37 [1.20, 4.70]
Subtotal	586	414		1.83 [1.30, 2.56]
Total events: 154 (treatment), 64 (control)				
(p = 0.57), I² = 0%				
Test for heterogeneity: χ² = 2.90, df = 4				
Test for overall effect: z = 3.49 (p = 0.0005)				
Risperidone studies				
Mahmoud et al. (28)	26/137	12/131		2.32 [1.12, 4.83]
Keitner et al. (30)	32/62	8/33		3.33 [1.30, 8.53]
Reeves et al. (29)	4/12	2/11		2.25 [0.32, 15.76]
Subtotal	211	175		2.63 [1.51, 4.57]
Total events: 62 (treatment), 22 (control)				
Test for heterogeneity: χ² = 0.38, df = 2				
(p = 0.83), I² = 0%				
Test for overall effect: z = 3.43 (p = 0.0006)				
Quetiapine studies				
Khullar et al. (31)	3/8	0/7		9.55 [0.40, 225.19]
Mattingly et al. (32)	11/24	2/13		4.65 [0.84, 25.66]
McIntyre et al. (33)	9/29	5/29		2.16 [0.62, 7.49]
Earley et al. (12)	110/327	38/160		1.63 [1.06, 2.50]
El-Khalili et al. (13)	112/289	35/143		1.95 [1.25, 3.06]
Subtotal	677	352		1.89 [1.41, 2.54]

Figure 5.2 Atypical antipsychotics (second-generation antipsychotics, SGAs) in treatment-resistant depression (TRD). Remission rates from a metaanalysis by Nelson & Papakostas (2009), reprinted with permission

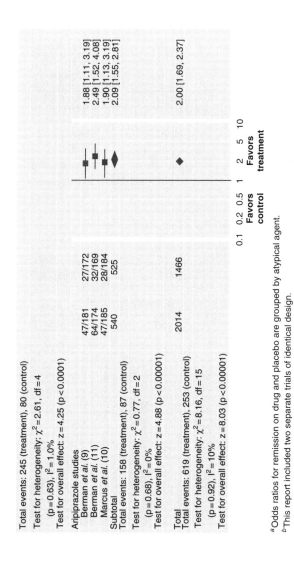

Total events: 245 (treatment), 80 (control)

Test for heterogeneity: $\chi^2 = 2.61$, df = 4
  (p = 0.63), $I^2 = 1.0\%$
Test for overall effect: z = 4.25 (p < 0.0001)

Aripiprazole studies
Berman et al. (9)   47/181   27/172   1.88 [1.11, 3.19]
Berman et al. (11)   64/174   32/169   2.49 [1.52, 4.08]
Marcus et al. (10)   47/185   28/184   1.90 [1.13, 3.19]
Subtotal   540   525   2.09 [1.55, 2.81]

Total events: 158 (treatment), 87 (control)

Test for heterogeneity: $\chi^2 = 0.77$, df = 2
  (p = 0.68), $I^2 = 0\%$
Test for overall effect: z = 4.88 (p < 0.00001)

Total   2014   1466   2.00 [1.69, 2.37]
Total events: 619 (treatment), 253 (control)

Test for heterogeneity: $\chi^2 = 8.16$, df = 15
  (p = 0.92), $I^2 = 10\%$
Test for overall effect: z = 8.03 (p < 0.00001)

0.1 0.2 0.5   1   2   5   10
     Favors   Favors
     control   treatment

[a]Odds ratios for remission on drug and placebo are grouped by atypical agent.
[b]This report included two separate trials of identical design.

Figure 5.2 (*Continued*)

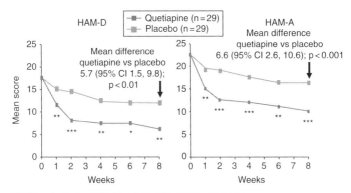

Figure 5.3 Effect on depression (HAM-D) and anxiety (HAM-A) ratings of quetiapine augmentation of SSRIs/SNRIs. McIntyre *et al.*, 2007

or placebo in addition to SSRIs or SNRIs. In both depression ratings, as measured by the Hamilton Total Score, and anxiety ratings, as measured by the Hamilton Anxiety Score, statistically significant differences were obtained at all time points. From a practical point of view, it is important to note that a differentiation between the placebo group and the quetiapine group was already apparent after 1 week, a finding that has also been confirmed by other authors (Bauer *et al.*, 2009; Konstantinidis *et al.*, 2012; Liebowitz *et al.*, 2010). These data would not have been achieved in a switching paradigm, nor with a combination of other antidepressants, with the exception of mirtazapine (Blier *et al.*, 2010).

Currently, quetiapine extended-release formulation is the only SGA approved for use in MDD in Europe. Its usage has been approved as an add-on medication to ongoing antidepressant treatment in patients with a suboptimal response to antidepressants (European Medicines Agency, 2011). Interestingly, in the USA aripiprazole is also indicated for the adjunctive treatment of MDD and olanzapine is indicated in combination with fluoxetine for treatment-resistant depression (TRD). As it stands right now, neither aripiprazole nor olanzapine will be granted this

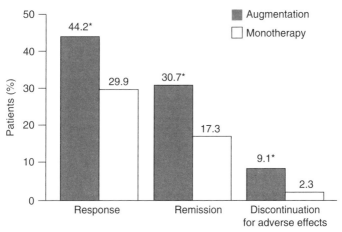

*p < 0.00001 vs. placebo

Figure 5.4 Atypical antipsychotic (second-generation antipsychotics, SGAs) augmentation in major depressive disorder (MDD): metaanalysis of 16 double-blind studies; rates of response, remission and discontinuation as a result of adverse events. Data from Papakostas & Fava (2009), published in Schlaepfer *et al.* (2012), reprinted with permission

indication from the EMA, since aripiprazole and olanzapine do not provide placebo-controlled long-term data, as required by the EMA. Furthermore, the EMA has a specific understanding that indication not be granted for a fixed combination, which stands for the olanzapine and fluoxetine combination.

Side effects

Side effects of SGAs stem from the varying degrees of $\alpha 1$ adrenergic (orthostatic hypotension), antihistaminergic (weight gain, sedation) or antimuscarinergic (cognitive dysfunction, dry mouth, constipation) activity of these agents.

Figure 5.4 depicts the favourable response and remission data obtained from the metaanalysis by Nelson & Papakostas

(2009). Additionally, this graph contains the discontinuation data for adverse events, which are about four times greater than those in antidepressant monotherapy. Based on the pharmacodynamic properties, it is therefore advisable to choose a medication which does not cause side effects considered to be bothersome by the patient, such as weight gain and constipation (Fava *et al.*, 2009).

Further notice should also be given to the interaction profile, in the sense that the addition of an SGA raises the level of the antipsychotic, with the occurrence of EPS side effects. This is apparent, for example, when risperidone is added to previously used fluoxetine: approximately a doubling of the level of risperidone can be expected, with the possible occurrence of EPS side effects.

Conclusions

Although the use of SGAs has now become an important part of everyday clinical practice for the treatment of depression (Klein *et al.*, 2004), several questions need to be addressed, as outlined in Box 5.1. Probably the most important point is that SGAs are not all the same (Hartung *et al.*, 2008; Stahl, 2000). They differ based on their pharmacodynamic properties, specifically with regard to the metabolic syndrome and the EPS side-effect profile (Kasper *et al.*, 2006). Data are also available for half-year administration of quetiapine for the indication of depression, but we do not have evidence for its long-term efficacy beyond this timespan. Depression is in most cases a life-long illness and therefore phase 4 data must be collected to establish this. Clinicians are also confronted with the possibility of lithium, T3 or antidepressant augmentation therapy. Based on the available literature, it needs to be stated that the database for placebo-controlled augmentation with SGAs is at least ten times larger than that for lithium or antidepressant augmentation, which on the other hand does not devaluate the findings of the latter. The algorithm determining when to use SGAs in the

---

Box 5.1   Questions to be addressed in augmentation with second-generation antipsychotics (SGAs) in depression

- Are all SGAs the same?
- Is there evidence for long-term efficacy?
- How does SGA augmentation compare with other augmentation strategies?
- How should clinicians use SGAs in their treatment algorithm (T3, Li, MAO-I, buspirone, mirtazapine)?
- Should dosing be lower than for mania or psychosis?
- Are there any side-effect concerns (EPS-TD, prolactin, metabolic syndrome)?

Table 5.4   Changes in conceptualizations of depression

Then	Now
Situational versus endogenous	*Interplay of biology and environment*
No known pathology, possible 'chemical imbalance'	Emerging evidence of cellular and brain-circuit pathology
High treatment response rates and full recovery as the rule	**Progressive** disorder with worse outcomes over time
Wait-and-see attitude; habit-based prescribing	Aggressive, individualized treatment, targeting **remission** is needed

treatment sequence has also not yet been specified and awaits further clarification. Given the rapid onset of action, the beneficial side-effect profile of most SGAs administered in low doses favours their use. Available studies include lower dosages used for mania or psychosis, and this seems to be common knowledge. Quetiapine 100–300 mg, olanzapine 5–10 mg, aripiprazole 5–10 mg, ziprasidone 40–80 mg and risperidone 1–3 mg are the preferred dosages.

Clinicians are well advised to monitor the side-effect profiles of the available medication, watching for higher EPS or tardive dyskinesia during the use of risperidone and the likelihood of a metabolic syndrome with olanzapine, for example. The latter is important if the antidepressant treatment applied before it includes the risk of a metabolic syndrome, as is the case for mirtazapine.

A new augmentation strategy obtained with the use of SGAs and other treatment modalities also delineates a change in the conceptualization of depression (see Table 5.4), which includes not only biological variables but also the interplay of biology and environment. Furthermore, a new understanding should include evidence of brain-circuit pathology and consider depression as a progressive disorder with a deteriorating outcome over time. Given this understanding, an intensive, individualized programme should be started, targeting remission. The appropriate use of SGAs is a promising option.

References

Bauer, M., Pretorius, H. W., Constant, E. L. *et al.* (2009) Extended-release quetiapine as adjunct to an antidepressant in patients with majore depressive disorder: results of a randomized, placebo-controlled, double-blind study. *J. Clin. Psychiatry*, **70**, 540–549.

Bauer, M., Bschor, T., Pfennig, A. *et al.* on behalf of the WFSBP Task Force on Treatment Guidelines for Unipolar Depressive Disorders (2007) World Federation of Societies of Biological Psychiatry (WFSBP) guidelines for biological treatment of unipolar depressive disorders in primary care. *World J. Biol. Psychiatry*, **8**, 67–104.

Berman, R. B., Fava, M., Thase, M. E. *et al.* (2008) The third consecutive, positive, double-blind, placebo controlled trial of aripiprazole augmentation in the treatment of major depression. *American College of Neuropsychopharmacology 2008 Annual Meeting Abstracts* (Scottsdale, AZ, December 7–11, 2008), ACNP, Nashville, TN, USA.

Berman, R. M., Marcus, R. N., Swanink, R. *et al.* (2007) The efficacy and safety of aripiprazole as adjunctive therapy in major depressive disorder: a multicenter, randomized, double-blind, placebo-controlled study. *J. Clin. Psychiatry*, **68**, 843–853.

Blier, P., Ward, H. E., Tremblay, P. *et al.* (2010) Combination of antidepressant medications from treatment. initiation for major depressive disorder: a double-blind randomized study. *Am. J. Psychiatry*, **167**, 281–288.

Chen, J., Gao, K. & Kemp, D. E. (2011) Second-generation antipsychotics in major depressive disorder? Update and clinical perspective. *Curr. Opin. Psychiatry*, **24**, 10–17.

Correll, C. U., Leucht, S. & Kane, J. M. (2004) Lower risk for tardive dyskinesia associated with second-generation antipsychotics: a systematic review of 1-year studies. *Am. J. Psychiatry*, **161**, 414–425.

Corya, S. A., Williamson, D. J., Sanger, T. M. *et al.* (2006) A randomized, double-blind comparison of olanzapine/fluoxetine combination, olanzapine, fluoxetine, and venlafaxine in treatment-resistant depression. *Depression & Anxiety*, **23**, 364–372.

Dunner, D. L., Amsterdam, J. D., Shelton, R. C. *et al.* (2007) Efficacy and tolerability of adjunctive ziprasidone in treatment-resistant depression: a randomized, open-label, pilot study. *J. Clin. Psychiatry*, **68**, 1071–1077.

Earley, W., McIntyre, A., Bauer, M. *et al.* (2007) Efficacy and tolerability of extended release quetiapine fumarate (quetiapine extended release) as add-on to antidepressants in patients with major depressive disorder (MDD): results from a double-blind, randomized, phase III study. *American College of Neuropsychopharmacology 2007 Annual Meeting Abstracts* (Boca Raton, FL, December 9–13, 2007), ACNP, Nashville, TN, USA.

El-Khalili, N., Joyce, M., Atkinson, S. *et al.* (2008) Adjunctive extended-release quetiapine fumarate (quetiapine-extended release) in patients with major depressive disorder and inadequate antidepressant response. *American Psychiatric Association 2008 Annual Meeting: New Research Abstracts* (Washington, DC, May 3–8, 2008), APA, Washington, DC, USA.

El-Khalili, N., Joyce, M., Atkinson, S. *et al.* (2010) Extended-release quetiapine fumarate (quetiapine XR) as adjunctive therapy in major depressive disorder (MDD) in patients with an inadequate response to ongoing antidepressant treatment: a multicentre, randomized, double-blind, placebo-controlled study. *Int. J. Neuropsychopharmacol.*, **13**, 917–932.

European Medicines Agency (2011) Seroquel XR. http://www.ema.europa.eu/ema/index.jsp?curl=pages/medicines/human/referrals/Seroquel_XR/human_referral_000206.jsp&mid=WC0b01ac0580024e9a, last accessed November 9, 2012.

Farah, A. (2005) Atypicality of atypical antipsychotics. *Prim. Care Comp.*, **7**, 268–274.

Fava, M. (2001) Augmentation and combination strategies in treatment-resistant depression. *J. Clin. Psychiatry*, **62**(Suppl.), 4–11.

Fava, M., Wisniewski, S. R., Thase, M. E. *et al.* (2009) Metabolic assessment of aripiprazole as adjunctive therapy in major depressive disorder: a pooled analysis of 2 studies. *J. Clin. Psychopharmacol.*, **29**, 362–367.

Goodwin, G., Fleischhacker, W., Arango, C. *et al.* (2009) Advantages and disadvantages of combination treatment with antipsychotics ECNP Consensus Meeting, March 2008, Nice. *Eur. Neuropsychopharmacol.*, **19**, 520–532.

Grohmann, R., Engel, R. R., Rüther, E. & Hippius, H. (2004) The AMSP Drug Safety Program: methods and global results. *Pharmacopsychiatry*, **37**(Suppl.), 4–11.

Hartung, D. M., Wisdom, J. P., Pollack, D. A. *et al.* (2008) Patterns of atypical antipsychotic subtherapeutic dosing among Oregon Medicaid patients. *J. Clin. Psychiatry*, **69**, 1540–1547.

Jensen, N. H., Rodriguiz, R. M., Caron, M. G. *et al.* (2008) N-desalkylquetiapine, a potent norepinephrine reuptake inhibitor and partial 5-HT1A agonist, as a putative mediator of quetiapine's antidepressant activity. *Neuropsychopharmacol.*, **33**, 2303–2312.

Kasper, S. (1998) How much do novel antipsychotics benefit the patients? *Int. Clin. Psychopharmacol.*, **13**(Suppl.), 71–77.

Kasper, S., Lowry, A., Hodge, A. *et al.* (2006) Tardive dyskinesia: analysis of outpatients with schizophrenia from Latin America, Asia, Central and Eastern Europe, and Africa and the Middle East. *Schiz. Res.*, **81**, 139–143.

Kaye, J. A., Bradbury, B. D. & Jick, H. (2003) Changes in antipsychotic drug prescribing by general practitioners in the United Kingdom from 1991 to 2000, a population-based observational study. *Brit. J. Clin. Pharmacol.*, **56**, 569–575.

Keitner, G. I., Garlow, S. J., Ryan, C. E. *et al.* (2009) A randomized, placebo-controlled trial of risperidone augmentation for patients with difficult-to-treat unipolar, non-psychotic major depression. *J. Psy. Res.*, **43**, 205–214.

Khullar, A., Chokka, P., Fullerton, D. *et al.* (2006) A double-blind, randomized, placebo-controlled study of quetiapine as augmentation therapy to SSRI/SNRI agents in the treatment of non-psychotic unipolar depression with residual symptoms. *American Psychiatric Association 2006 Annual Meeting: New Research Abstracts* (Toronto, Canada, May 20–25, 2006), APA Washington, DC, USA.

Klein, N., Sacher, J., Wallner, H. *et al.* (2004) Therapy of treatment resistant depression: focus on the management of TRD with atypical antipsychotics. *CNS Spectrum*, **9**, 823–832.

Konstantinidis, A., Hrubos, W., Nirnberger, G. *et al.* (2007) Quetiapine in combination with citalopram in patients with unipolar psychotic depression. *Prog. Neuropsychopharmacol. Biol. Psychiatry*, **31**, 242–247.

Konstantinidis, A., Papageorgiou, K., Grohmann, R. *et al.* (2012) Increase of antipsychotic medication in depressive inpatients from 2000 to 2007: results from the AMSP International Pharmacovigilance Program. *Int. J. Neuropsychopharmacol.*, **15**, 449–457.

Lenderts, S. & Kalali, A. (2009) Treatment of depression: an update on antidepressant monotherapy and combination therapy. *Psychiatry*, **6**, 15–17.

Liebowitz, M., Lam, R. W., Lepola, U. *et al.* (2010) Efficacy and tolerability of extended release quetiapine fumarate monotherapy as maintenance treatment of major depressive disorder: a randomized, placebo-controlled trial. *Depression & Anxiety*, **27**, 964–976.

Mahmoud, R. A., Pandina, G., Turkoz, I. *et al.* (2007) Risperidone for treatment-refractory major depressive disorder. *Ann. Int. Med.*, **147**, 593–602.

Marcus, R., McQuade, R., Carson, W. *et al.* (2008) The efficacy and safety of aripiprazole as adjunctive therapy in major depressive disorder: a second multicenter, randomized, double-blind placebo-controlled study. *J. Clin. Psychopharmacol.*, **28**, 156–165.

Mattingly, G., Ilivicky, H., Canale, J. & Anderson, R. (2006) Quetiapine combination for treatment-resistant depression. *American Psychiatric Association 2006 Annual Meeting: New Research Abstracts* (Toronto, Canada, May 20–25, 2006), APA, Washington, DC, USA.

McIntyre, A., Gendron, A. & McIntyre, A. (2007) Quetiapine adjunct to selective serotonin reuptake inhibitors or venlafaxine in patients with major depression, comorbid anxiety, and residual depressive symptoms: a randomized, placebo-controlled pilot study. *Depression & Anxiety*, **24**, 487–494.

Mohamed, S., Leslie, D. L. & Rosenheck, R. A. (2009) Use of antipsychotics in the treatment of major depressive disorder in the U.S. Department of Veterans Affairs. *J. Clin. Psychiatry*, **70**, 906–912.

Nelson, J. C. (1987) The use of antipsychotic drugs in the treatment of depression, in *Treating Resistant Depression* (ed. J. Zohar & R. H. Belmaker), PMA Publishing, New York, NY, pp. 131–146.

Nelson, J. C. & Papakostas, G. I. (2009) Atypical antipsychotic augmentation in major depressive disorder: a meta-analysis of placebo-controlled randomized trials. *Am. J. Psychiatry*, **166**, 980–991.

Olfson, M. & Marcus, S. C. (2009) National patterns in antidepressant medication treatment. *Arch. Gen. Psychiatry*, **66**, 848–856.

Ostroff, R. B. & Nelson, J. C. (1999) Risperidone augmentation of selective serotonin reuptake inhibitors in major depression. *J. Clin. Psychiatry*, **60**, 256–259.

Papakostas, G. I., Shelton, R. C., Smith, J. & Fava, M. (2007) Augmentation of antidepressants with atypical antipsychotic medications for treatment-resistant major depressive disorder: a meta-analysis. *J. Clin. Psychiatry*, **68**, 826–831.

Philip, N. S., Carpenter, L. L., Tyrka, A. R. & Price, L. H. (2008) Augmentation of antidepressants with atypical antipsychotics: a review of the current literature. *J. Psy. Pract.*, **14**, 34–44.

Philip, N. S., Carpenter, L. L., Tyrka, A. R. & Price, L. H. (2010) Pharmacologic approaches to treatment resistant depression: a re-examination for the modern era. *Exp. Op. Pharacother.*, **11**, 709–722.

Reeves, H., Batra, S., May, R. S. *et al.* (2008) Efficacy of risperidone augmentation to antidepressant in the management of suicidality in major depressive disorder: a randomized, double-blind, placebo controlled pilot study. *J. Clin. Psychiatry*, **69**, 1228–1336.

Reynolds, G. P. (2004) Receptor mechanisms in the treatment of schizophrenia. *J. Psychopharmacol.*, **18**, 340–345.

Rush, A. J., Trivedi, M. H., Wisniewski, S. R. *et al.* (2006) Acute and longer-term outcomes in depressed outpatients requiring one or several treatment steps: a STAR*D report. *Am. J. Psychiatry*, **163**, 1905–1917.

Schläpfer, T., Agren, H., Monteleone, P. *et al.* (2012) The hidden third: improving outcome in treatment resistant depression. *J. Psychopharmacol.*, **26**, 587–602.

Shelton, R. C. & Papakostas, G. I. (2008) Augmentation of antidepressants with atypical antipsychotics for treatment-resistant major depressive disorder. *Acta Psychiatr. Scand.*, **117**, 253–259.

Shelton, R. C., Tollefson, G. D., Tohen, M. *et al.* (2001) A novel augmentation strategy for treating resistant major depression. *Am. J. Psychiatry*, **158**, 131–134.

Shelton, R. C., Williamson, D. J., Corya, S. A. *et al.* (2005) Olanzapine/ fluoxetine combination for treatment-resistant depression: a controlled study of SSRI and nortriptyline resistance. *J. Clin. Psychiatry*, **66**, 1289–1297.

Stahl, M. (2000) *Essential Psychopharmacology: Neuroscientific Basis and Practical Applications*, Cambridge University Press, Cambridge, UK.

Stahl, S. M. & Shayegan, D. K. (2003) The psychopharmacology of ziprasidone: receptor-binding properties and real-world psychiatric practice. *J. Clin. Psychiatry*, **64**(Suppl. 19), 6–12.

Tadori, Y., Forbes, R. A., McQuade, R. D. & Kikuchi, T. (2008) Characterization of aripiprazole partial agonist activity at human dopamine D(3) receptors. *Eur. J. Pharmacol.*, **597**, 27–33.

Tatsumi, M., Jansen, K., Blakely, R. D. & Richelson, E. (1999) Pharmacologic profile of neuroleptics at human monoamine transporters. *Eur. J. Pharmacol.*, **368**, 277–283.

Thase, M., Corya, S. A., Osuntokun, O. *et al.* (2007) A randomized, double-blind comparison of olanzapine/fluoxetine combination, olanzapine, and fluoxetine in treatment-resistant major depressive disorder. *J. Clin. Psychiatry*, **68**, 224–236.

Wheeler Vega, J. A., Mortimer, A. M. & Tyson, P. J. (2003) Conventional antipsychotic prescription in unipolar depression, I: an audit and recommendations for practice. *J. Clin. Psychiatry*, **64**, 568–574.

Zhang, W., Perry, K. W., Wong, D. T. *et al.* (2000) Synergistic effects of olanzapine and other antipsychotic agents in combination with fluoxetine on norepinephrine and dopamine release in rat prefrontal cortex. *Neuropsychopharmacol.*, **23**, 250–262.

CHAPTER 6

Lithium, Thyroid Hormones and Further Augmentation Strategies in Treatment-resistant Depression

Robert Haußmann and Michael Bauer

Department of Psychiatry and Psychotherapy, University Hospital Carl Gustav Carus, Dresden University of Technology, Dresden, Germany

Summary

A variety of pharmacologically different nonantidepressant agents have been studied for their ability to augment the efficacy of antidepressants in depressed patients who do not respond sufficiently. Among the strategies reviewed in this chapter, augmentation with lithium is the best-evidenced, showing clear efficacy in a metaanalysis of 10 placebo-controlled trials. All other commonly used augmentation strategies described in this chapter are not well supported by sufficient data from randomized controlled trials (RCTs). There is also a lack of controlled comparator studies with different augmentation agents.

Treatment-resistant Depression, First Edition. Edited by Siegfried Kasper and Stuart Montgomery.
© 2013 John Wiley & Sons, Ltd. Published 2013 by John Wiley & Sons, Ltd.

Such studies are needed to better guide physicians in the treatment of nonresponders to standard antidepressants.

Introduction

Major depressive disorder (MDD) is a severe disabling condition that requires effective treatment to reduce symptoms and improve quality of life. However, MDD continues to be a major concern in clinical practice as antidepressant treatment is not effective at achieving an adequate initial response in a relatively large proportion of patients and is often associated with a delayed onset of therapeutic efficacy. Regardless of the initial choice of antidepressant, about 30–50% of patients with a major depressive episode will not respond sufficiently to adequately performed first-line treatment (Bauer *et al.*, 2007).

Various alternative treatment strategies have been proposed for non- or partially responsive depressions in MDD. Possible treatment strategies for patients with a depressive episode who are nonresponsive to an adequate trial of any antidepressant include:

- a dose adjustment;
- the addition of a second antidepressant (combination therapy of two antidepressants);
- the introduction of another drug not itself considered an antidepressant (augmentation or adjunct treatment);
- a switch to an alternative antidepressant (monotherapy).

The option of augmentation treatment is believed to have some advantages. One is that it eliminates the period of transition between one antidepressant and another and builds on the partial response. Consequently, when it works, an augmentation strategy can be rapidly effective. Another advantage is that patients who have had some response may be reluctant to risk losing that improvement; in such situations, augmentation may be beneficial.

A variety of options have been studied with regard to augmenting antidepressant treatment, including lithium, atypical antipsychotics, anticonvulsants, psychostimulants and the thyroid hormones. These are all reviewed in this chapter, with the exception of the atypical antipsychotics (which is discussed in Chapter 5). Table 6.1 summarizes the major pharmacological augmentation strategies and presents the documented empirical evidence for their efficacy.

Augmentation studies

Lithium

Augmentation with lithium is among the best-evidenced augmentation therapies available for depressed patients who do not respond to standard antidepressants. Lithium salts have been used to augment the efficacy of antidepressant medications for more than 30 years (Bschor *et al.*, 2007). The first study to test their use in patients with MDD was performed by de Montigny *et al.* (1981), who reported a dramatic response within 48 hours of the addition of lithium in eight patients who had not responded to at least 3 weeks of treatment with tricyclic antidepressants. The efficacy of the combination and rapidity of response has led many clinical research groups to pursue study of this treatment intervention. Subsequent randomized controlled trials (RCTs) have confirmed de Montigny's initial findings, with more than 30 open-label and comparator studies that included more than 500 depressed patients being published (Bauer *et al.*, 2010). In these studies, the duration of antidepressant pretreatment ranged between 3 and 7 weeks, with a mean of 4.5 weeks; the subsequent lithium augmentation therapy lasted between 2 days and 14 weeks, with a mean duration of about 30 days. The antidepressants used in the trials included agents from different groups, among them selective serotonin reuptake inhibitors (SSRIs), tri- and tetracyclic antidepressants and monoamine oxidase inhibitors (MAOIs).

Table 6.1 Pharmacological augmentation strategies in major depressive disorder (MDD)

Class	Individual agent	Dose range	Main mechanism of action	Level of evidence[a]	Reference
Lithium salts		0.5–0.7 mmol/l[b]	Mood stabilizer	A	Bauer & Döpfmer (1999), Bauer et al. (2010), Crossley et al. (2007)
Atypical antipsychotics	Aripiprazole	5–15 mg/day	Dopamine (D2)- and serotonin (5-HT1A)-receptor partial agonist, serotonin (5-HT2A) antagonist	A	See Chapter 5
	Quetiapine	150–300 mg/day	Serotonin (5-HT2A)- and dopamine (D2)-receptor antagonist	A	See Chapter 5
Thyroid hormones	Triiodothyronine (T3)	25–50 µg/day	Thyroid hormone	B	Aronson et al. (1996)
	Levothyroxine (L-T4)	200–400 µg/day	Thyroid hormone	C	Bauer et al. (1998, 2005)

Anticonvulsants	Lamotrigine	50–500 mg/day	Mood stabilizer/anticonvulsant	C	Barbee & Jamhour (2002), Barbee et al. (2011), Barbosa et al. (2003), Carvalho et al. (2007), Ivkovic et al. (2009), Thomas et al. (2010)
	Carbamazepine	200–1200 mg/day, 20–40 µmol/l	Mood stabilizer/anticonvulsant	C	Ciusani et al. (2004), Otani et al. (1996), Schüle et al. (2009), Steinacher et al. (2002)
	Valproic acid	600 mg/day	Mood stabilizer/anticonvulsant	C	Fang et al. (2011)
Dopamine agonists	Bromocriptine	7.5–52.5 mg/day	Dopamine (D2)-receptor agonist	C	Bouras & Bridges (1982), Carvalho et al. (2007), Colonna et al. (1979), Inoue et al. (1996), Theohar et al. (1982)
	Pergolide	0.25–2.0 mg/day	Dopamine (D1/D2)-receptor agonist	C	Bouckoms & Mangini (1993), Carvalho et al. (2007), Izumi et al. (2000)

(Continued)

Table 6.1 (Continued)

Class	Individual agent	Dose range	Main mechanism of action	Level of evidence[a]	Reference
	Pramipexole	0.375–1.0 mg/day	Dopamine (D2/D3)-receptor agonist	C	Carvalho et al. (2007), Lattanzi et al. (2002)
Psychostimulants	Methylphenidate	18–80 mg/day	Facilitating effect on dopaminergic and noradrenergic neurotransmission	C	Carvalho et al. (2007), DeBattista et al. (2003), Patkar et al. (2006), Ravindran et al. (2008)
	Modafinil	100–400 mg/day	Facilitating effect on dopaminergic and noradrenergic neurotransmission	C	Abolfazli et al. (2011), Carvalho et al. (2007), Dunlop et al. (2007), Fava et al. (2005)
Buspirone		10–60 mg/day	Partial 5-hydroxytryptamine$_{1A}$ (5-HT1A) receptor agonist	C	Carvalho et al. (2007)

Pindolol		7.5 mg/day	Beta-adrenoreceptor/5-HT1A-receptorantagonist	C	Bressa (1994), Carvalho et al. (2007)
Nutrition supplements					
Omega-3-polyunsaturated fatty acids	Eicosapentaenoic acid	0.6–4.0 g/day	Nutritional supplement	C	Lesperance et al. (2001), Nemets et al. (2002), Silvers et al. (2004)
	Docosahexaenoic acid	2.4 g/day	Nutritional supplement	C	Lesperance et al. (2001)
S-Adenosyl-Methionine		1600 g/day	Nutritional supplement	C	Yehuda et al. (1998)

[a] Level A–D, classification modified from WFSBP guidelines (Bauer et al., 2007), where A = good evidence from randomized controlled trials (RCTs), B = moderate evidence from RCTs, C = low evidence from RCTs, D = no evidence.
[b] Serum level.

The dosages of the antidepressants used were not reported in all trials; the dosages of lithium carbonate ranged between 300 and 1500 mg/day. The response rates ranged widely between 23.5 and 100%, with a median of 56%; 10 of 17 open studies found response rates to lithium augmentation of 50% or more.

A metaanalysis addressing the efficacy of lithium augmentation therapy pooled 10 randomized, double-blind, placebo-controlled trials and included 269 mostly unipolar depressed patients (Crossley & Bauer, 2007). Lithium had a significant positive effect versus placebo, with an odds ratio of 3.11, which corresponds to a number needed to treat (NNT) of 5. The metaanalysis revealed a mean response rate of 41.2% in the lithium group and 14.4% in the placebo group. One placebo-controlled trial in the continuation treatment phase showed that responders to acute-phase lithium augmentation should be maintained on the lithium–antidepressant combination for at least 12 months in order to prevent early relapses (Bauer *et al.*, 2000; Bschor *et al.*, 2002).

However, five of the acute studies pooled did not show a significant difference. Reasons for the negative findings might be low power (Browne *et al.*, 1990; Kantor *et al.*, 1986; Zusky *et al.*, 1988), use of insufficient lithium doses (Stein & Bernadt, 1993), too short duration of treatment (Browne *et al.*, 1990; Kantor *et al.*, 1986) or concerns about the efficacy of lithium augmentation with noradrenergic antidepressants (Bschor & Bauer, 2004; Nierenberg *et al.*, 2003). Previous studies had demonstrated that only doses of lithium carbonate higher than 600 mg/day and a duration of 7 or more days were efficacious (Bauer & Döpfmer, 1999). As noted in the earlier metaanalysis from 1999 (Bauer & Döpfmer, 1999), a new negative study would have to include more than 2500 patients per group in order to change the results of this pooling.

Still, it remains to be examined whether the response to lithium augmentation represents true augmentation resulting from synergistic effects or is simply due to the antidepressant effect of lithium itself. There is some experimental evidence supporting the former possibility (reviewed in Bauer *et al.*, 2010). From the clinical point of view, arguments for a true augmentation effect derive from a controlled clinical trial showing that the antidepressant effect of lithium addition was significantly higher in amitriptyline-pretreated depression patients compared with placebo-pretreated patients, who showed no improvement after a 3-week treatment (de Montigny *et al.*, 1983). In summary, a randomized, double-blind study that investigates the effects of lithium alone and compares them with the effects of lithium in combination with an anti-depressant is warranted.

In clinical practice, a relatively fast titration regimen can be administered (in people aged 55 or younger: dose of lithium carbonate day $1 = 450$ mg, day $2 = 900$ mg) without major adverse effects, in order to achieve optimal plasma lithium serum levels (0.5 and 0.7 mmol/l).

Thyroid hormones

The evidence that thyroid hormones are essential to the normal development of the brain and to the prevalence of behavioural and neuropsychiatric symptoms in thyroid disease, especially the disturbances of affect found in hypothyroidism (Whybrow & Bauer, 2005), have long suggested an intimate relationship between thyroid hormone metabolism and mood disorder (Bauer *et al.*, 2008). Individuals who suffer mood disorder frequently have disturbed indices of peripheral thyroid function, and clinical studies extending over 3 decades suggest that thyroid hormones can modulate the expression of both unipolar and bipolar disease when used in conjunction with psychotropic agents.

In contrast, efforts to employ thyroid hormones *alone* as therapeutic agents in mood disorder and other psychiatric illnesses have rarely been successful (Flach *et al.*, 1958). Nonetheless, since Prange's classic acceleration studies in the late 1960s using triiodothyronine, T_3, in association with the tricyclic antidepressant imipramine (Prange *et al.*, 1958), a series of open and controlled clinical trials have confirmed the adjunctive therapeutic value of thyroid hormones. Specifically, there is some evidence that T_3 (dose range: 25–50 mcg/day) may augment the response to antidepressants in treatment-resistant depressed (TRD) patients, although here the results have been inconsistent (Aronson *et al.*, 1996; Cooper-Kazaz *et al.*, 2007).

Since then, in a series of open-label studies, adjunctive treatment with supraphysiological doses of levothyroxine, L-T$_4$, have shown effective and well tolerated in the maintenance treatment of patients suffering the malignant phenotype of rapid cycling and in otherwise prophylaxis-resistant bipolar disorders (Bauer & Whybrow, 1990; Bauer *et al.*, 2002a; Baumgartner *et al.*, 1994). Augmentation with supraphysiological doses of L-T$_4$ has also been reported to have immediate therapeutic value in antidepressant-resistant bipolar and unipolar depressed patients during a phase of refractory depression (Bauer *et al.*, 1998, 2005). In these studies of severely ill and treatment-refractory patients, an aggregate of approximately two-thirds of individuals experience significant improvement from affective symptoms (and women benefit more from the thyroid hormone supplementation than do men). As we have gained more experience with the use of supraphysiological doses of L-T$_4$ in patients with refractory mood disorder, however, it has become apparent that many patients who respond to the adjunctive treatment have serum thyroid hormone levels within normal limits and give no past history of peripheral thyroid disease. In our own practice, we find that patients with refractory affective disorders tolerate high doses of L-T$_4$ surprisingly well, and in follow-up studies over an extended period we have observed few adverse effects from the induced hyperthyroxinaemia (Bauer *et al.*, 1998, 2004; Ricken *et al.*, 2012). This low incidence of harmful side effects, including upon bone mineral density, as well as the high tolerability, contrasts with the response typically seen in patients with primary thyroid disease who are receiving high-dose thyroid hormone therapy. For example, patients with thyroid carcinoma treated with high doses of L-T$_4$ in order to achieve suppression of thyroid-stimulating hormone (TSH) commonly complain of the symptoms of thyrotoxicosis.

Supplementing standard treatment regimens with thyroid hormone must still be considered an experimental therapeutic approach in affective disorders. Due to limited evidence from controlled data and potential hazards, treatment with supraphysiological doses of L-T$_4$ (dose range: 200–400 mcg/day) should be reserved to patients with *refractory* mood disorder.

Anticonvulsants

Several antiepileptic drugs have been tested in augmentation therapy of TRD recently (Barbee *et al.*, 2011; Ciusani *et al.*, 2004; Fang *et al.*, 2011; Ivkovic *et al.*, 2009; Schüle *et al.*, 2009). Most are well known as mood stabilizers in bipolar disorders (e.g. lamotrigine, carbamazepine and valproic acid) (Yatham *et al.*, 2005, 2006). Considering the number and quality of studies conducted within the last couple of years, lamotrigine might be the best-tested anticonvulsant in augmenting antidepressants (Barbee & Jamhour, 2002; Barbee *et al.*, 2011; Barbosa *et al.*, 2003; Ivkovic *et al.*, 2009; Gabriel, 2006; Gutierrez *et al.*, 2005).

There have been some trials and chart reviews to suggest the efficacy of lamotrigine in ameliorating depressive symptoms in patients suffering from TRD when it is used as an augmenting agent in concomitant treatment with antidepressants (Barbosa *et al.*, 2003; Gabriel, 2006; Gutierrez *et al.*, 2005). Unfortunately, the data published to date demonstrate only little evidence to recommend the use of lamotrigine in augmentation of TRD. Large RCTs are needed so we can learn more about the antidepressive efficacy of lamotrigine as an augmenting agent (Thomas *et al.*, 2010).

Several open-label trials, retrospective chart reviews and case series have focused on the antidepressive potential of carbamazepine (Dietrich & Emrich, 1998; Wunderlich *et al.*, 1982, 1983). A few of these mainly concentrated on the role of carbamazepine as an augmenting agent in antidepressive medication (Ciusani *et al.*, 2004; Otani *et al.*, 1996; Schüle *et al.*, 2009; Steinacher *et al.*, 2002). In animal models, it has been demonstrated that carbamazepine leads to an increase of serotonin in the brain (Dailey *et al.*, 1998).

When being used in augmentation therapy, carbamazepine causes a metabolic induction of the concomitantly given antidepressant, which can lead to reduced plasma concentration levels of antidepressive agents (Ciusani *et al.*, 2004; Otani *et al.*, 1996; Schüle *et al.*, 2009; Steinacher *et al.*, 2002). This represents a well-known finding in antidepressive augmentation therapy with carbamazepine (Leinonen *et al.*, 1991), although its clinical relevance still needs to be demonstrated in larger studies (Schüle *et al.*, 2009). In general, the trials conducted suggest a limited efficacy of carbamazepine in augmenting antidepressive therapy. Moreover, a recently published open-label study could not reproduce the antidepressant efficacy of carbamazepine in augmentation therapy with mirtazapine (Schüle *et al.*, 2009).

As early as 1996, an open study reported the efficacy of valproic acid in patients with unipolar depression (Davis *et al.*, 1996). In a very recently published pilot study, valproic acid was shown to be effective in TRD in a Chinese population. In this study the valproic acid group had higher remission rates than four other augmentation strategies (Fang *et al.*, 2011). Although these findings need to be reproduced in other ethnic groups and in larger placebo-controlled trials, valproic acid had been reviewed as an effective treatment of MDD previously (Vigo & Baldessarini, 2009). To our knowledge there are no placebo-controlled trials on the use of valproic acid in the augmentation of TRD to date. Therefore, further large and placebo-controlled trials are needed to evaluate the potential of valproic acid as an augmenting agent in this indication.

Despite the finding that phenytoin seems to be as potent as fluoxetine in the treatment of unipolar disorder (Nemets *et al.*, 2005), there is no evidence of an augmenting efficacy (Shapira *et al.*, 2006).

Dopamine agonists

The neurobiology of depressive disorders is based on dys-functional noradrenaline, serotonin and dopamine systems (Nierenberg *et al.*, 1998). A new generation of antidepressive agents such as venlafaxine and bupropion inhibits the presyn-aptic dopamine uptake (Lemke, 2006). Patients suffering from severe depression with psychomotor slowing are known to have a reduced dopamine turnover (Roy *et al.*, 1992). Surprisingly, L-dopa *per se* does not seem to have an antidepressant effect (Goodwin *et al.*, 1970; Pare & Sandler, 1959). Since dopamine agonists harbour an antidepressive effect, the augmentation of antidepressants by dopamine agonists by definition represents a combination therapy for some authors (Lemke, 2006).

In the late 1970s an uncontrolled pilot study showed a limited response in depressed patients treated with bromocrop-tine monotherapy (Colonna *et al.*, 1979). The antidepressive properties of bromocriptine have been further tested in various uncontrolled and controlled studies, where a similar antide-pressive potential comparable to that of amitriptyline and imi-pramine was demonstrated (Bouras & Bridges, 1982; Theohar *et al.*, 1982). Bromocriptine was also shown to be efficient in antidepressive augmentation of tricyclic and heterocyclic anti-depressants in a preliminary open study (Inoue *et al.*, 1996).

Pergolide, a mixed D1/D2 dopamine-receptor agonist, can also be an efficient adjunctive drug to augment antidepressive medication when used in combination with both tricyclic anti-depressants and MAOIs, whereas it has no antidepressant effect when administered alone (Bouckoms & Mangini, 1993). Furthermore, pergolide was tested in TRD, added to tricyclic and heterocyclic antidepressants. In this preliminary open study, approximately 40% of patients greatly improved, suggesting a role for dopamine-receptor stimulation (Izumi *et al.*, 2000).

The most recently tested dopamine-receptor agonist in aug-mentation strategies is the D2/D3 dopamine-receptor agonist pramipexole, which was tested in unipolar depressed patients responding to either tricyclic antidepressants or SSRIs. This naturalistic prospective study of the efficacy of pramipexole adjunctive therapy in TRD suggested some evidence for this approach (Lattanzi *et al.*, 2002).

In conclusion, more controlled research data to clarify the role of dopamine-receptor agonists in augmenting antidepressants are clearly needed.

Psychostimulants

Psychostimulants are known to have a significant facilitating effect on dopaminergic and noradrenergic neurotransmission and have been tested in numerous studies as an augmentation option in combination with commonly used antidepressants such as tricyclic antidepressants, MAOIs, SSRIs and serotonin norepinephrine reuptake inhibitors (SNRIs) (Bauer *et al.*, 2002b; Carvalho *et al.*, 2007; Fawcett *et al.*, 1991; Feighner *et al.*, 1985; Linet, 1989; Masand *et al.*, 1998; Metz & Shader, 1991; Stoll *et al.*, 1996; Wharton *et al.*, 1971). A recently published literature review concerning these studies summarized efficacy issues regarding the role of psychostimulants in TRD (Carvalho *et al.*, 2007). Although the data obtained suggested an efficacy for psychostimulants in TRD, the relatively short half-life of these substances continues to be a major drawback (Bourin *et al.*, 1995).

Recently, Patkar *et al.* (2006) published a 4-week, randomized, double-blind, placebo-controlled trial studying the efficacy and tolerability of augmentation therapy with methylphenidate in patients suffering from TRD. In this study, no statistically significant benefit was demonstrated. Even more recently, another double-blind, randomized, placebo-controlled trial testing for the augmentative capacity of an osmotic-release oral methylphenidate system was published; again, this study showed no significant effect on depressive symptoms. However, a reduction of apathy and fatigue symptoms was achieved by adjunctive treatment with methylphenidate in this latter study (Ravindran *et al.*, 2008).

Several studies have looked at the use of another stimulant, modafinil, for adjunctive treatment in depressive disorders. One of these placebo-controlled studies evaluated the effects of modafinil on fatigue and sleepiness in patients partially responding to ongoing antidepressant therapy. Compared to placebo, the modafinil group improved significantly with regard to fatigue and wakefulness. This advantage of modafinil over placebo was no longer present at week 6 of treatment (DeBattista *et al.*, 2003). Fava *et al.* (2005) conducted a controlled trial testing the potential of modafinil augmentation in partial SSRI responders. This study indicated effective augmention efficacy of modafinil in severely depressed patients. Dunlop *et al.* (2007) published a double-blind, placebo-controlled study adding modafinil or placebo to SSRI. This trial did not show beneficial effects of modafinil on symptoms of depression. Very recently, the augmentation therapy of modafinil and fluoxetine has been shown to be superior to that of fluoxetine and placebo when examining overall depression levels and remission rates (Abolfazli *et al.*, 2011). Against this background, modafinil seems to be an effective augmenting agent in treating TRD, although further validation is needed (Carvalho *et al.*, 2007, 2008).

Buspirone

Buspirone is a partial agonist at the postsynaptic 5-HT1A receptor. It enhances the activity of SSRIs via this receptor (Redrobe & Bourin, 2008).

In 1993 an open study of buspirone augmentation of serotonin reuptake inhibitors in refractory depression suggested that buspirone might be useful in patients not responding to SSRI treatment (Joffe & Schuller, 1993). In 1998 the first double-blind, placebo-controlled, randomized trial testing buspirone in addition to an SSRI in the treatment of TRD was published. This trial showed no superiority of buspirone compared to a placebo regimen (Landen *et al.*, 1998). A further placebo-controlled, randomized, double-blind trial examining buspirone augmentation of citalopram or fluoxetine showed a significantly greater reduction of depressive symptoms in the buspirone group. The authors concluded that patients with severe depressive symptoms may benefit from buspirone augmentation (Appelberg *et al.*, 2001).

The augmentation therapy of buspirone plus citalopram was shown to have a similar efficacy to the combination therapy of bupropione and citalopram concerning remission rates, though combination therapy led to fewer side effects (Trivedi *et al.*, 2006). In a recently published pilot study comparing five different augmentation strategies, buspirone augmentation was proved to be similarly effective to risperidone, valproate, trazodone and thyroid hormone regimens (Fang *et al.*, 2011).

In summary, as reviewed by Carvalho *et al.* (2008), the 'ultimate evidence' for the efficacy of buspirone in TRD still needs to be determined.

S-Adenosyl methionine

S-adenosyl methionine (SAMe) is a naturally occurring methyl donor in human metabolism. Its highest concentrations can be measured in the liver, adrenal glands and pineal gland (Bottiglieri, 2002). In 1994 a metaanalysis of clinical trials studying SAMe as an antidepressant showed its superiority to placebo and a comparable antidepressive effect to that of tricyclic antidepressive agents (Bressa, 1994). Very recently, SAMe was tested for the amelioration of depressive symptoms in augmentation therapy with SSRIs. This double-blind, controlled trial could not show a significantly relevant effect but suggested the usefulness of SAMe in antidepressive augmentation (Papakostas *et al.*, 2010). In order to evaluate the augmentative antidepressive potential of SAMe in TRD, further study is needed.

Omega-3 polyunsaturated fatty acids

Fatty acids harbour multiple functions regarding central nervous system (CNS) metabolism. They are known to have a variety of biological influences on neurochemical systems, being much more than a simple source of energy (Yehuda *et al.*, 1998). In the mid-1990s, Hibbeln & Salem (1995) described a low incidence of depressive disorders in fish oil-consuming countries.

Omega-3 polyunsaturated fatty acids (PUFAs) have been tested in augmentation studies in TRD. Eicosapentaenoic acid (EPA) and docosahexaenoic acid (DHA) are the most examined PUFAs concerning their augmentative potential in combination with antidepressants. Peet & Horrobin (2002) conducted a dose-ranging study into the augmentative effects of EPA in patients with ongoing depression despite adequate treatment with antidepressants. EPA was tested at dosages of 1, 2 and 4 g. In this study, EPA was added for 12 weeks to the previously given antidepressants, which mainly consisted of SSRIs and tricyclic antidepressants. There was a significantly better outcome in the 1 g EPA group compared to the placebo group, while this observation was not evident at the other dosages. In another study, conducted by Nemets *et al.* (2002), EPA was tested in augmentation of antidepressive medication (SSRIs) for 3 weeks at a dose of 2 g. A significant benefit was shown in the EPA group compared to placebo. Furthermore, a randomized, double-blind, placebo-controlled trial (Silvers *et al.*, 2004) left doubts concerning the efficacy of omega-3 fatty acids in the treatment of depression. In this study, 8 g fish oil consisting of 0.6 g EPA and 2.4 g DHA was not shown to be effective in ameliorating depressive symptoms compared to control. In one further trial, only a tendency towards superiority of omega-3 fatty acids over placebo was detected (Lesperance *et al.*, 2011). Recently, a critical metaanalysis of randomized, placebo-controlled trials of omega-3 fatty acid treatment of depression, as either augmentation or monotherapy, questioned positive study results, remarking that almost all data suggesting the efficacy of fatty acids might be due to publication bias (Bloch & Hannestad, 2011). Although the efficacy of omega-3 fatty acids as an augmenting medication in depressive patients has been questioned recently, there are some studies suggesting beneficial effects.

Combined treatment with antidepressants from the beginning: acceleration studies

When considering therapeutic aspects of TRD, it is crucial to differentiate between augmentation and acceleration regarding antidepressant efficacy. In addition to the high rates of nonresponders to treatment with standard antidepressants, the delayed onset of therapeutic response remains another major clinical dilemma. Substantial benefits typically do not become evident until 2–3 weeks after the initiation of treatment with any of the currently available antidepressants. Reducing this latency time would markedly reduce the suffering and impairment associated with depression.

Against this background, several medications have been tested concerning their acceleration efficacy of antidepressants. Specifically, a number of studies with different agents not considered antidepressants (e.g. lithium, triiodothyronine, pindolol, PUFAs) have assessed whether the use of a medication prescribed initially with antidepressants speeds the response time to antidepressants (so-called *acceleration studies*) in patients with major depression.

Lithium

Five randomized, double-blind, placebo-controlled trials assessing the effect of concomitant administration of lithium and antidepressant (tri- and tetracyclics) on response time in the acute treatment phase of depression (total 231 participants) have been included in a metaanalysis (Crossley & Bauer, 2007).

A modest evidence for lithium's acceleration of response to antidepressants was found (standardized mean difference of −0.43, 95% CI = −0.93 to 0.07).

Triiodothyronine

A metaanalysis supports the efficacy of triiodothyronine (T_3) in accelerating clinical response to tricyclic antidepressants in a population of nonrefractory depressed patients (Altshuler *et al.*, 2001): five of the six studies included found triiodothyronine to be significantly more effective than placebo in accelerating clinical response, demonstrating a pooled, weighted effect size index (d) of 0.58 (95% CI, 0.21–0.94) and a significant average effect (z = 3.10, p = 0.002). Furthermore, the effects of T_3 acceleration were greater as the percentage of women participating in the study increased.

Pindolol

Pindolol, a ß-adrenoreceptor/5-HT1A-receptor antagonist, has been shown to accelerate the antidepressant action of SSRIs in a double-blind, randomized, placebo-controlled trial testing the augmentative efficacy of pindolol treatment with clomipramine, fluoxetine, fluvoxamine or paroxetine in TRD (Perez *et al.*, 1999). As there were contradictory results concerning the role of pindolol in acceleration, Ballesteros & Callado (2004) conducted a metaanalysis analysing its capacity to hasten the antidepressive effect of SSRIs within nine RCTs. In this analysis, the authors came to the conclusion that pindolol accelerates the antidepressive effect within the first weeks of treatment.

Beyond these trials, pindolol has been separately tested in combination with paroxetine in depressed inpatients who were not previously treated. Again, significant effects were demonstrated (Geretsegger *et al.*, 2007). In combination with venlafaxine, the acceleration potential seems to depend on the metabolic capacity of the patient, which might potentially give an explanation for former contradictory study results concerning pindolol's acceleration efficacy (Martiny *et al.*, 2012).

Polyunsaturated fatty acids

In 2009 an RCT analysed the acceleration efficacy of omega-3 fatty acids given concomitantly with 50 mg of sertraline. Patients were treated with 930 mg EPA and 750 mg DHA. The study could not demonstrate any superiority of combination treatment over sertraline monotherapy (Carney *et al.*, 2009). Very recently, omega-3 fatty acids where also tested in combination with citalopram. Despite higher dosages compared with previous studies (1800 mg EPA and 400 mg DHA), no enhanced speed of response was observed. Nevertheless, the combination therapy of EPA and DHA with citalopram was superior to citalopram monotherapy regarding the effectiveness in decreasing symptoms of depression (Gertsik *et al.*, 2012).

Conclusions

A variety of pharmacologically different nonantidepressant agents have been studied for their ability to augment the efficacy of antidepressants in depressed patients who were not responding sufficiently to treatment. Among the strategies reviewed in this chapter, augmentation with lithium is the best-evidenced augmentation therapy, showing clear efficacy in a metaanalysis of 10 placebo-controlled trials. All other commonly used augmentation strategies described here are not well supported by sufficient data from RCTs. There is also a lack of controlled comparator studies with different augmentation agents; such studies are needed to better guide physicians in the treatment of nonresponders to standard antidepressants.

References

Abolfazli, R., Hosseini, M., Ghanizadeh, A. *et al.* (2011) Double-blind randomized parallel-group clinical trial of efficacy of the combination fluoxetine plus modafinil versus fluoxetine plus placebo in the treatment of major depression. *Depression & Anxiety*, **28**, 297–302.

Altshuler, L. L., Bauer, M., Frye, M. A. *et al.* (2001) Does thyroid supplementation accelerate tricyclic antidepressant response? A review and meta-analysis of the literature. *Am. J. Psychiatry*, **158**, 1617–1622.

Appelberg, B. G., Syvälahti, E. K., Koskinen, T. E. *et al.* (2001) Patients with severe depression may benefit from buspirone augmentation of selective serotonin reuptake inhibitors: results from a placebo-controlled, randomized, double-blind, placebo wash-in study. *J. Clin. Psychiatry*, **62**(6), 448–452.

Aronson, R., Offman, H. J., Joffe, R. T. *et al.* (1996) Triiodothyronine augmentation in the treatment of refractory depression. A meta-analysis. *Arch. Gen. Psychiatry*, **53**, 842–848.

Ballesteros, J. & Callado, L. (2004) Effectiveness of pindolol plus serotonin uptake inhibitors in depression: a meta-analysis of early and late outcomes from randomized controlled trials. *J. Affect. Disord.*, **79**, 137–147.

Barbee, J. & Jamhour, N. (2002) Lamotrigine as an augmentation agent in treatment-resistant depression. *J. Clin. Psychiatry*, **63**(8), 737–741.

Barbee, J. G., Thompson, T. R., Jamhour, N. J. *et al.* (2011) A double-blind placebo-controlled trial of lamotrigine as an antidepressant augmentation agent in treatment-refractory unipolar depression. *J. Clin. Psychiatry*, **72**(10), 1405–1412.

Barbosa, L., Berk, M. & Vorster, M. (2003) A double-blind, randomized, placebo-controlled trial of augmentation with lamotrigine or placebo in patients concomitantly treated with fluoxetine for resistant major depressive episodes. *J. Clin. Psychiatry*, **64**(4), 403–407.

Bauer, M. & Döpfmer, S. (1999) Lithium augmentation in treatment-resistant depression: meta-analysis of placebo-controlled studies. *J. Clin. Psychopharmacol.*, **19**, 427–434.

Bauer, M. S. & Whybrow, P. C. (1990) Rapid cycling bipolar affective disorder. II. Treatment of refractory rapid cycling with high-dose levothyroxine: a preliminary study. *Arch. Gen. Psychiatry*, **47**, 435–440.

Bauer, M., Hellweg, R., Graf, K. J. & Baumgartner, A. (1998) Treatment of refractory depression with high-dose thyroxine. *Neuropsychopharmacol.*, **18**, 444–455.

Bauer, M., Bschor, T., Kunz, D. *et al.* (2000) Double-blind, placebo-controlled trial of the use of lithium to augment antidepressant medication in continuation treatment of unipolar major depression. *Am. J. Psychiatry*, **157**(9), 1429–1435.

Bauer, M., Berghofer, A., Bschor, T. *et al.* (2002a) Supraphysiological doses of L-thyroxine in the maintenance treatment of prophylaxis-resistant affective disorders. *Neuropsychopharmacol.*, **27**, 620–628.

Bauer, M., Whybrow, P. C., Angst, J. *et al.* (2002b) World Federation of Societies of Biological Psychiatry (WFSBP) guidelines for biological treatment of unipolar depressive disorders, part 1: acute and continuation treatment of major depressive disorder. *World J. Biol. Psychiatry*, **3**, 5–43.

Bauer, M., Fairbanks, L., Berghofer, A. *et al.* (2004) Bone mineral density during maintenance treatment with supraphysiological doses of levothyroxine in affective disorders: a longitudinal study. *J. Affect. Disord.*, **83**, 183–190.

Bauer, M., London, E. D., Rasgon, N. *et al.* (2005) Supraphysiological doses of levothyroxine alter regional cerebral metabolism and improve mood in women with bipolar depression. *Mol. Psychiatry*, **10**, 456–469.

Bauer, M., Bschor, T., Pfenning, A. *et al.* (2007) World Federation of Societies of Biological Psychiatry (WFSBP) guidelines for biological treatment of unipolar depressive disorders in primary care. *World J. Biol. Psychiatry*, **8**, 67–104.

Bauer, M., Goetz, T., Glenn, T. & Whybrow, P. C. (2008) The thyroid-brain interaction in thyroid disorders and mood disorders. *J. Neuroendocrinol.*, **20**, 1101–1114.

Bauer, M., Adli, M., Bshcor, T. *et al.* (2010) Lithium's emerging role in the treatment of refractory major depressive episodes: augmentation of antidepressants. *Neuropsychobiol.*, **62**, 36–44.

Baumgartner, A., Bauer, M. & Hellweg, R. (1994) Treatment of intractable non-rapid cycling bipolar affective disorder with high-dose thyroxine: an open clinical trial. *Neuropsychopharmacol.*, **10**, 183–189.

Bloch, M. H. & Hannestad, J. (2011) Omega-3 fatty acids for the treatment of depression: systematic review and meta-analysis. *Mol. Psychiatry*, doi:10.1038/mp.2011.100.

Bottiglieri, T. (2002) S-adenosyl-l-methionine (SAMe), from the bench to the bedside: molecular basis of a pleiotropic molecule. *Am. J. Clin. Nutr.*, **75**, 1151S–1157S.

Bouckoms, A. & Mangini, L. (1993) Pergolide: an antidepressant adjuvant for mood disorders? *Psychopharmacol. Bull.*, **29**(2), 207–211.

Bouras, N. & Bridges, P. (1982) Bromocriptine and depression. *Curr. Med. Res. Opin.*, **8**, 150–153.

Bourin, M., Le Melledo, J. & Malinge, M. (1995) Experimental and clinical pharmacology of psychostimulant. *Can. J. Psychiatry*, **40**, 401–410.

Bressa, G. (1994) S-adenosyl-methionine (SAMe) as antidepressant: meta-analysis of clinical studies. *Acta Neurol. Scand. Suppl.*, **154**, 7–14.

Browne, M., Lapierre, Y. D., Hrdina, P. D. & Horn, E. (1990) Lithium as an adjunct in the treatment of major depression. *Int. Clin. Psychopharmacol.*, **5**(2), 103–110.

Bschor, T. & Bauer, M. (2004) Is successful lithium augmentation limited to serotonergic antidepressants? *J. Clin. Psychopharmacol.*, **24**, 240–241.

Bschor, T., Berghofer, A., Strohle, A. *et al.* (2002) How long should the lithium augmentation strategy be maintained? A 1-year follow-up of a placebo-controlled study in unipolar refractory major depression. *J. Clin. Psychopharmacol.*, **22**, 427–430.

Bschor, T., Lewitzka, U., Pfennig, A. *et al.* (2007) Fünfundzwanzig Jahre Lithiumaugmentation. *Nervenarzt*, **78**, 1237–1247.

Carney, R., Freedland, K. E., Rubin, E. H. *et al.* (2009) Omega-3 augmentation of sertraline in treatment of depression in patients with coronary heart disease. *JAMA*, **302**(15), 1651–1657.

Carvalho, A., Cavalcante, J. L., Castelo, M. S. & Lima, M. C. O. (2007) Augmentation strategies for treatment-resistant depression: a literature review. *J. Clin. Pharm. Ther.*, **32**, 415–428.

Carvalho, A., Machado, J. & Cavalcante, J. (2008) Augmentation strategies for treatment-resistant depression. *Curr. Opin. Psychiatry*, **22**, 7–12.

Ciusani, E., Zullino, D. F., Eap, C. B. *et al.* (2004) Combination therapy with venlafaxine and carbamazepine in depressive patients not responding to venlafaxine: pharmakokinetic and clinical aspects. *J. Psychopharmacol.*, **18**(4), 559–566.

Colonna, L., Petit, M. & Lepine, J. (1979) Bromocriptine in affective disorders. A pilot study. *J. Affect. Disord.*, **1**(3), 173–177.

Cooper-Kazaz, R., Apter, J. T., Cohen, R. *et al.* (2007) Combined treatment with sertraline and liothyronine in major depression: a randomized, double-blind, placebo-controlled trial. *Arch. Gen. Psychiatry*, **64**, 679–688.

Crossley, N. A. & Bauer, M. (2007) Acceleration and augmentation of antidepressants with lithium for depressive disorders: two meta-analyses of randomized, placebo-controlled trials. *J. Clin. Psychiatry*, **68**, 935–940.

Dailey, J., Reith, M. E., Steidley, K. R. *et al.* (1998) Carbamazepine-induced release of serotonin from rat hippocampus in vitro. *Epilepsia*, **39**(10), 1054–1063.

Davis, L., Kabel, D., Patel, D. *et al.* (1996) Valproate as an antidepressant in major depressive disorder. *Psychopharmacol. Bull.*, **32**(4), 647–652.

DeBattista, C., Doghramji, K., Menza, M. A. *et al.* (2003) Adjunct modafinil for the short-term treatment of fatigue and sleepiness in patients with major depressive disorder: a preliminary double-blind, placebo-controlled study. *J. Clin. Psychiatry*, **64**, 1057–1064.

de Montigny, C., Grunberg, F., Mayer, A. *et al.* (1981) Lithium induces rapid relief of depression in tricyclic antidepressant drug non-responders. *Brit. J. Psychiatry*, **138**, 252–256.

de Montigny, C., Cournoyer, G., Morissette, R. *et al.* (1983) Lithium carbonate neurobiologic actions of tricyclic antidepressant drugs and lithium ion on the serotonin system. *Arch. Gen. Psychiatry*, **40**(12), 1327–1334.

Dietrich, D. & Emrich, H. (1998) The use of anticonvulsants to augment antidepressant medication. *J. Clin. Psychiatry*, **59**(Suppl. 5), 51–58.

Dunlop, B. W., Crits-Christoph, P., Evans, D. L. *et al.* (2007) Coadministration of modafinil and a selective serotonin reuptake inhibitor from the initiation of treatment of major depressive disorder with fatigue and sleepiness: a double-blind, placebo-controlled study. *J. Clin. Psychopharmacol.*, **27**(6), 614–619.

Fang, Y., Yuan, C., Xu, Y. *et al.* (2011) A pilot study of the efficacy and safety of paroxetine augmented with risperidone, valproate, buspirone, trazodone, or thyroid hormone in adult Chinese patients with treatment-resistant major depression. *J. Clin. Psychopharmacol.*, **31**(5), 638–642.

Fava, M., Thase, M. & DeBattista, C. (2006) A multicenter, placebo-controlled study of modafinil augmentation in partial responders to selective serotonin reuptake inhibitors with persistent fatigue and sleepiness. *J. Clin. Psychiatry*, **66**, 85–93.

Fawcett, J., Kravitz, H. M., Zajecka, J. M. *et al.* (1991) CNS stimulant potentiation of monoamine oxidase inhibitors in treatment-refractory depression. *J. Clin. Psychopharmacol.*, **11**, 127–132.

Feighner, J., Herbstein, J. & Damlouji, N. (1985) Combined MAOI, TCA and direct stimulant therapy of treatment-resistant depression. *J. Clin. Psychiatry*, **46**, 206–209.

Flach, F. F., Celian, C. I. & Rawson, R. W. (1958) Treatment of psychiatric disorders with triiodothyronine. *Am. J. Psychiatry*, **114**, 841–842.

Gabriel, A. (2006) Brief report: lamotrigine adjunctive treatment in resistant unipolar depression: an open, descriptive study. *Depression & Anxiety*, **23**, 485–488.

Geretsegger, C., Bitterlich, W., Stelzig, R. *et al.* (2007) Paroxetine with pindolol augmentation: a double-blind, randomized, placebo-controlled study in depressed in-patients. *Eur. Neuropsychopharmacol.*, **18**, 141–146.

Gertsik, L., Poland, R., Bresee, C. *et al.* (2012) Omega-3 fatty acid augmentation of citalopram treatment for patients with major depressive disorder. *J. Clin. Psychopharmacol.*, **32**(1), 61–64.

Goodwin, F. K., Post, R. M., Dunner, D. L. *et al.* (1970) L-Dopa, catecholamines and behaviour – a clinical and biochemical study in depressed patients. *Biol. Psychiatry*, **2**(4), 341–366.

Gutierrez, R., McKercher, R., Galea, J. & Jamison, K. L. (2005) Lamotrigine augmentation strategy for patients with treatment-resistant depression. *CNS Spectrum*, **10**(10), 800–805.

Hibbeln, J. & Salem, N. J. (1995) Dietary polyunsaturated fatty acids and depression: when cholesterol does not satisfy. *Am. J. Clin. Nutr.*, **62**, 1–9.

Inoue, T., Tsuchiya, K., Miura, J. *et al.* (1996) Bromocriptine treatment of tricyclic and heterocyclic antidepressant-resistant depression. *Biol. Psychiatry*, **40**, 151–153.

Ivković, M., Damjanović, A., Jovanović, A. *et al.* (2009) Lamotrigine versus lithium augmentation of antidepressant therapy in treatment-resistant depression: efficacy and tolerability. *Psychiatr. Danub.*, **21**(2), 187–193.

Izumi, T., Inoue, T., Kitagawa, N. *et al.* (2000) Open pergolide treatment of tricyclic and heterocyclic antidepressant-resistant depression. *J. Affect. Disord.*, **61**, 127–132.

Joffe, R. & Schuller, D. (1993) An open study of buspirone augmentation of serotonin reuptake inhibitors in refractory depression. *J. Clin. Psychiatry*, **54**(7), 269–271.

Kantor, D., McNevin, S., Leichner, P. *et al.* (1986) The benefit of lithium carbonate adjunct in refractory depression – fact or fiction? *Can. J. Psychiatry*, **31**(5), 416–418.

Landen, M., Bjorling, G., Agren, H. & Fahlen, T. (1998) A randomized, double-blind, placebo-controlled trial of buspirone in combination with an SSRI in patients with treatment-refractory depression. *J. Clin. Psychiatry*, **59**(12), 664–668.

Lattanzi, L., Dell'Osso, L., Cassano, P. *et al.* (2002) Pramipexole in treatment-resistant depression: a 16-week naturalistic study. *Bipolar Disord.*, **4**(5), 307–314.

Leinonen, E., Lillsunde, P., Laukkanen, V. *et al.* (1991) Effects of carbamazepine on serum antidepressant concentrations in psychiatric patients. *J. Clin. Psychopharmacol.*, **11**, 313–325.

Lemke, M. (2006) Dopaminagonisten als Antidepressiva – experimentelle und klinische Befunde. *Nervenarzt*, **78**, 31–38.

Lesperance, F., Frasure-Smith, N., St-André, E. *et al.* (2011) The efficacy of omega-3 supplementation for major depression: a randomized controlled trial. *J. Clin. Psychiatry*, **72**(8), 1054–1062.

Linet, L. (1989) Treatment of a refractory depression with a combination of fluoxetine and d-amphetamine. *Am. J. Psychiatry*, **146**(6), 803–804.

Martiny, K., Lunde, M., Bech, P. & Plenge, P. (2012) A short-term double-blind randomized controlled pilot trial with active or placebo pindolol in patients treated with venlafaxine for major depression. *Nord. J. Psychiatry*, **66**, 147–154.

Masand, P., Anand, V. & Tanquary, J. (1998) Psychostimulant augmentation of second generation antidepressants: a case series. *Depression & Anxiety*, **7**, 89–91.

Metz, A. & Shader, R. (1991) Combination of fluoxetine with pemoline in the treatment of major depressive disorder. *Int. Clin. Psychopharmacol.*, **6**(2), 93–96.

Nemets, B., Stahl, Z. & Belmaker, R. (2002) Addition of omega-3 fatty acid to maintenance medication treatment for recurrent unipolar depressive disorder. *Am. J. Psychiatry*, **159**, 477–479.

Nemets, B., Bersudsky, Y. & Belmaker, R. (2005) Controlled double-blind trial of phenytoin vs. fluoxetine in major depressive disorder. *J. Clin. Psychiatry*, **66**, 586–590.

Nierenberg, A., Dougherty, D. & Rosenbaum, J. (1998) Dopaminergic agents and stimulants as an antidepressant augmentation strategies. *J. Clin. Psychiatry*, **59**(Suppl. 5), 60–63.

Nierenberg, A. A., Papakostas, G. I., Petersen, T. *et al.* (2003) Lithium augmentation of nortriptyline for subjects resistant to multiple antidepressants. *J. Clin. Psychopharmacol.*, **23**(1), 92–95.

Otani, K., Yasui, N., Kaneko, S. *et al.* (1996) Carbamazepine augmentation therapy in three patients with trazodone-resistant unipolar depression. *Int. Clin. Psychopharmacol.*, **11**(1), 55–57.

Papakostas, G. I., Mischoulon, D., Shyu, I. *et al.* (2010) S-adenosyl methionine (SAMe) augmentation of serotonin reuptake inhibitors for antidepressant non-responders with major depressive disorder: a double-blind, randomized clinical trial. *Am. J. Psychiatry*, **167**(8), 942–948.

Pare, C. & Sandler, M. (1959) A clinical and biochemical study of a trial of iproniazid in the treatment of depression. *J. Neurol. Neurosurg. Psychiatry*, **22**, 247–251.

Patkar, A., Masand, P. S., Pae, C. U. *et al.* (2006) A randomized, double-blind, placebo-controlled trial of augmentation with an extended release formulation of methylphenidate in outpatients with treatment-resistant depression. *J. Clin. Psychopharmacol.*, **26**(6), 653–656.

Peet, M. & Horrobin, D. (2002) A dose-ranging study of the effects of ethyl-eicosapentaenoate in patients with ongoing depression despite apparently adequate treatment with standard drugs. *Arch. Gen. Psychiatry*, **59**, 913–919.

Perez, V., Soler, J., Puigdemont, D. *et al.* (1999) A double-blind, randomized, placebo-controlled trial of pindolol augmentation in depressive patients resistant to serotonin reuptake inhibitors. *Arch. Gen. Psychiatry*, **56**, 375–379.

Prange, A. J. Jr, Wilson, I. C., Rabon, A. M. & Lipton, M. A. (1969) Enhancement of imipramine antidepressant activity by thyroid hormone. *Am. J. Psychiatry*, **126**, 457–469.

Ravindran, A., Kennedy, S. H., O'Donovan, M. C. *et al.* (2008) Osmotic-release oral system methylphenidate augmentation of antidepressant monotherapy in major depressive disorder: results of a double-blind, randomized, placebo-controlled trial. *J. Clin. Psychiatry*, **69**(1), 87–94.

Redrobe, J. & Bourin, M. (1998) Dose-dependent influence of buspirone on the activities of selective serotonin reuptake inhibitors in the mouse forced swimming test. *Psychopharmacol.*, **138**, 198–206.

Ricken, R., Bermpohl, F., Schlattmann, P. *et al*. (2012) Long-term treatment with supraphysiological doses of thyroid hormone in affective disorders – effects on bone mineral density. *J. Affect. Disord.*, **136**(1–2), e89–94.

Roy, A., Karoum, F. & Pollack, S. (1992) Marked reduction in indexes of dopamine metabolism among patients with depression who attempt suicide. *Arch. Gen. Psychiatry*, **49**, 447–450.

Schüle, C., Baghai, T. C., Eser, D. *et al*. (2009) Lithium but not carbamazepine augments antidepressant efficacy of mirtazapine in unipolar depression: an open-label study. *World J. Biol. Psychiatry*, **10**(4), 390–399.

Shapira, B., Nemets, B., Trachtenberg, A. *et al*. (2006) Phenytoin as an augmentation for SSRI failures: a small controlled study. *J. Affect. Disord.*, **96**, 123–126.

Silvers, K. M., Woolley, C. C., Hamilton, F. C. *et al*. (2004) Randomised double-blind placebo-controlled trial of fish oil in the treatment of depression. *Prostaglandins Leukot. Essent. Fatty Acids*, **72**(3), 211–218.

Stein, G. & Bernadt, M. (1993) Lithium augmentation therapy in tricyclic-resistant depression. A controlled trial using lithium in low and normal doses. *Brit. J. Psychiatry*, **162**, 634–640.

Steinacher, L., Vandel, P., Zullino, D. F. *et al*. (2002) Carbamazepine augmentation in depressive patients non-responding to citalopram: a pharmacokinetic and clinical pilot study. *Eur. Neuropsychopharmacol.*, **12**(3), 255–260.

Stoll, A., Pillay, S. S., Diamond, L. *et al*. (1996) Methylphenidate augmentation of serotonine selective reuptake inhibitors: a case series. *J. Clin. Psychiatry*, **5**, 72–76.

Theohar, C., Fischer-Cornelssen, K., Brosch, H. *et al*. (1982) A comparative, multicenter trial between bromocriptine and amitriptyline in the treatment of endogenous depression. *Arzneimittelforschung*, **32**, 783–787.

Thomas, S., Nandhra, H. & Jayaraman, A. (2010) Systematic review of lamotrigine augmentation of treatment resistant unipolar depression (TRD). *J. Ment. Health*, **19**(2), 168–175.

Trivedi, M. H., Fava, M., Wisniewski, S. R. *et al*. (2006) Medication augmentation after the failure of SSRIs for depression. *N. Engl. J. Med.*, **354**(12), 1243–1252.

Vigo, D. & Baldessarini, R. (2009) Anticonvulsants in the treatment of major depressive disorder: an overview. *Harvard Rev. Psychiatry*, **17**, 231–241.

Wharton, R. N., Perel, J. M., Dayton, P. G. & Malitz, S. (1971) A potential clinical use for methylphenidate with tricyclic antidepressants. *Am. J. Psychiatry*, **127**, 1619–1625.

Whybrow, P. C. & Bauer, M. (2005) Behavioral and psychiatric aspects of hypothyroidism, in *Werner & Ingbar's The Thyroid. A Fundamental and Clinical Text*, 9th edition (ed. L. E. Braverman & R. D. Utiger), Lippincott Williams & Wilkins, Philadelphia, PA, USA, pp. 842–849.

Wunderlich, H., Heim, H. & Wunderlich, H. (1982) Carbamazepin (Finlepsin) bei endogenen affektiven Psychosen: eine neue Therapie. *Medicamentum*, **60**, 2–8.

Wunderlich, H., Grünes, J. U., Neumann, J. & Zahlten, W. (1983) Antidepressive therapy with carbamazepine (Finlepsin). *Arch. Neurol. Neurochir. Psychiatry*, **133**, 363–71.

Yehuda, S., Rabinovitz, S., Carasso, R. L. & Mostofsky, D. I. (1998) Fatty acids and brain peptides. *Peptides*, **19**(2), 407–419.

Yatham, L. N., Kennedy, S. H., O'Donovan, C. *et al.* (2005) Canadian Network for Mood and Anxiety Treatments (CANMAT) guidelines for the management of patients with bipolar disorder: consensus and controversies. *Bipolar Disord.*, **7**(Suppl. 3), 5–69.

Yatham, L. N., Kennedy, S. H., O'Donovan, C. *et al.* (2007) Canadian Network for Mood and Anxiety Treatments (CANMAT) guidelines for the management of patients with bipolar disorder: update 2007. *Bipolar Disord.*, **8**, 721–739.

Zusky, P. M., Biederman, J., Rosenbaum, J. F. *et al.* (1988) Adjunct low dose lithium carbonate in treatment-resistant depression: a placebo-controlled study. *J. Clin. Psychopharmacol.*, **8**(2), 120–124.

CHAPTER 7

The Role of Nonpharmacological Interventions in Treatment-resistant Depression

Thomas E. Schläpfer

*Department of Psychiatry and Psychotherapy,
University Hospital Bonn, Bonn, Germany; The Johns
Hopkins University School of Medicine, Maryland, USA*

Sarah Kayser

*Department of Psychiatry and Psychotherapy,
University Hospital Bonn, Bonn, Germany*

Summary

In approximately 50% of patients suffering from major depressive disorder (MDD), first-line antidepressant treatment is ineffective, and in about 30% of MDD patients, even four treatment steps yield insufficient antidepressant response. Stimulation of the human cerebral cortex with electrical currents was first described in 1874. In 1938, electroconvulsive therapy (ECT)

Treatment-resistant Depression, First Edition. Edited by Siegfried Kasper
and Stuart Montgomery.
© 2013 John Wiley & Sons, Ltd. Published 2013 by John Wiley & Sons, Ltd.

was first used for the treatment of depression and about 50 years later transcranial magnetic stimulation (TMS) for the same purpose was successfully accomplished. Today, ECT is established as one of the main columns in treatment-resistant depression (TRD) therapy. However, due to cognitive side effects and stigmatization, ECT is often used as a treatment of last resort. In recent years, novel techniques using electrical and magnetic fields to stimulate the brain have been developed. This chapter examines the use of ECT, TMS, vagus nerve stimulation (VNS), deep-brain stimulation (DBS) and magnetic seizure therapy (MST).

Introduction

In approximately 50% of patients suffering from major MDD, first-line antidepressant treatment is ineffective, and in about 30% of MDD patients, even four treatment steps yield no antidepressant response (Bartholow, 1874; Cerletti & Bini, 1938). Stimulation of the human cerebral cortex with electrical currents was first described in 1874 (Bartholow, 1874). In 1938, electroconvulsive therapy (ECT) was first used (Cerletti & Bini, 1938) and about 50 years later TMS was successfully accomplished (Barker *et al.*, 1985). In the years since, novel techniques using electrical and magnetic fields to stimulate the brain have been developed. This chapter examines the use of ECT, TMS, VNS, DBS and MST.

Electroconvulsive therapy

In 1938, the Italian psychiatrists Ugo Cerletti and Lucio Bini introduced ECT as a treatment for psychosis. Today, ECT is recognized as a routine treatment for severe depression, due to its antidepressant effect (70–90%) (Sackheim *et al.*, 2000) and fast onset of action (Lisanby, 2007). There are several guidelines for the application and performance of ECT (Abrams, 2002; Baghai *et al.*, 2004; Scott, 2004; Fink, 2009).

Indications, contraindications and risks

The primary indication of ECT is TRD (UK ECT Review Group, 2003), especially if there is a vital threat, such as suicidality, refusal of food and drink or delusional ideas (American Psychiatric Association & Weiner, 2001). Given the severity of psychiatric disorders such as TRD, there is no contraindication to the use of ECT, which is today a very safe treatment, whose risks are limited to common anaesthesia risks (mortality 1 : 50 000).

Mechanism of action

The mechanism of action is not yet fully understood. Modulation of the release of neurotransmitters (serotonin, noradrenalin and dopamine) has been proven (Wahlund & von Rosen, 2003) and there are hints of normalization of glutamate–glutamine metabolism (Pfleiderer *et al.*, 2003). Cortical gamma aminobutyric acid (GABA) concentration has been found to be increased after ECT (Mervaala *et al.*, 2001). The hypothesis of neuroplasticity supposes that there is an increase of glutamate junctions and neurogenesis following ECT, along with increases of brain-derived neurotrophic factor (BDNF), neurotrophin-3 (NT-3), nerve growth factor (NGF), glial cell-derived neurotrophic factor (GDNF) and fibroblast growth factor 2 (FGF2). Single photon-emission computed tomography (SPECT) studies have detected an increase of blood flow in the right temporal lobe and bilateral at the parietal cortex (Mervaala *et al.*, 2001). Additionally, a downmodulation of the hypothalamic–pituitary–adrenal (HPA) axis has been found over a course of ECT (Young *et al.*, 1990). Postictal suppression and the inhibitory regulation on the brain are probably responsible for the antidepressant effect. The induced seizures are secondary generalized, with an excitatory and inhibitory period. The duration of the seizure, the ictal and intraictal activity, the synchronicity, the propagation and the amplitude height are predictors of the therapeutic effect (Sackheim, 1999).

Procedure and stimulation parameters

Seizures are elicited under general anaesthesia with intravenous propofol, methohexital or thiopental as anaesthetics and intravenous succinylcholine as muscle relaxant. During the full course of anaesthesia, patients are oxygenated with 100% O_2. A rubber bite block must be inserted to prevent dental damage. The right leg is cuffed prior to the administration of the muscle relaxant and the duration of motor seizure activity is monitored by the cuffed-ankle method. Two channels of electroencephalogram (EEG) are usually recorded from frontal and mastoid electrodes. The physiological parameters, such as electrocardiogram (ECG) and blood pressure, are monitored during anaesthesia. The length of the full treatment is about 15 minutes. ECT treatments are not painful or inconvenient for the patient. Usually, Thymatron devices (specifically, Thymatron IV; Somatics Inc., USA) are used. The stimulation parameters are as follows: waveform bipolar, brief pulse current, square wave, frequency 10–70 Hz depending on the energy set (100–200 J or 504–1008 mC), pulse width 0.5 ms (0.25–1.0 ms), duration of stimulation 0.5–8.0 s. The standard electrode placements are right unilateral (RUL), left unilateral (LUL), bitemporal and bifrontal (American Psychiatric Association & Weiner, 2001) (see Figure 7.1). Bitemporal stimulation is useful for delusional depression, but today it is not established. There are three methods by which to determine the seizure threshold: the titration method, the high-dose method and the age method. The most common is the titration method (McCall *et al.*, 2000). For unilateral stimulation, a 2.5–6.0-fold seizure threshold is recommended; for bilateral stiumulation, 1.5–2.0-fold is suggested (Sackheim *et al.*, 1993). Commonly, a full ECT treatment course encompasses 10–12 sessions. The relapse rate after successful ECT is over 50% (Sackheim *et al.*, 2001). A maintenance ECT should be administered in some cases.

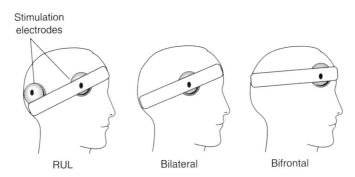

Stimulation
electrodes

RUL   Bilateral   Bifrontal

Figure 7.1 Standard electrode positions during electroconvulsive therapy (ECT). The three standard positions are: RUL (right unilateral – placed on the electrode frontotemporal)/LUL (left unilateral – not illustrated; placed on the electrode occipital); bilateral (bitemporal – an electrode placed on either side of the head, temporal); and bifrontal (an electrode placed on either side of the head, frontal)

Side effects

Acute side effects are transient anterograde amnesic deficits, cardiac and pulmonary complications, headache (20–40%), muscle pains, nausea (33%), postictal delirium (1–2%), neurological diseases (aphasia, agnosia and apraxia) and, extremely rarely, prolonged seizure or *status epilepticus*. Long-term side effects up to 30% are retrograde amnesic deficits (autobiographic memory).

Outlook

Ultrabrief pulse stimulation

The pulse width of ultrabrief pulse stimulation varies between 0.25 and 0.30 ms. A study with a frequency of 40 Hz and RUL stimulation over the seizure threshold demonstrated an antidepressant effect with less cognitive side effects than bilateral

ECT (Roepke *et al.*, 2011). Normally more than 12 treatments are required for a full course.

Focally electrically administered seizure therapy

Focally electrically administered seizure therapy (FEAST) combines a unidirectional stimulation with control of the polarity and an asymmetric electrode configuration (a small anterior and a large posterior electrode). The result is a lower seizure threshold compared to bilateral ECT (Spellman *et al.*, 2009).

Repetitive transcranial magnetic stimulation

Since 1985, TMS has been used for cortical stimulation. In 2008, the US Food and Drug Administration (FDA) approved repetitive transcranial magnetic stimulation (rTMS) for use in moderate TRD (O'Reardon *et al.*, 2007).

Indications, contraindications and risk

There is an evidence-based medicine (EBM) level I for rTMS in unipolar depression and moderate depression (exclusive or as an add-on combination with medication). More than 35 placebo-controlled studies have looked at rTMS, but the results are moderate concerning its antidepressant effect. The first long-term TMS study showed an antidepressant effect of 84% of patients over 24 weeks of TMS treatments (Janicak *et al.*, 2010). Contraindications are magnetic metal pieces in the head (except in the oral cavity), hearing implants and implanted medicine devices. Moderate contraindications are epileptic proneness and increased intracranial pressure. Cognitive functions are not affected after rTMS treatment (Janicak *et al.*, 2008); immediately following rTMS, patients can drive a car or return to work.

Mechanism of action

The antidepressant effect of rTMS has been associated with metabolism in the dorsolateral prefrontal cortex (DLPFC) (Nobler *et al.*, 2001). Many first-line rTMS studies reported relevant antidepressant effects after treatment (George *et al.*, 2000). However, further studies have somewhat reduced this result (Herwig *et al.*, 2007). The exact mechanism of action of rTMS is not yet fully understood. The TMS concept is based on modulation of the excitability of the brain and the role of circumscribed cortical regions and their associated areas. Further, changes in metabolism are seen after TMS at the anterior cingulate cortex (ACC) (Paus *et al.*, 2001), supplementary motor area (Siebner *et al.*, 1998), medial frontal cortex (Hayward *et al.*, 2007) and striatum (Pogarell *et al.*, 2007). Depending on the frequency, TMS can have different effects on the brain: a frequency <1 Hz induces inhibition (Hoffman & Cavus, 2002), while a high frequency (5–20 Hz) induces excitation (Ziemann *et al.*, 2008). rTMS also has an effect on the dopamine distribution in subcortical areas (Keck *et al.*, 2002) and on monoaminergic neurotransmission (Siebner *et al.*, 2003). In addition, there is a difference between acute and long-term effects. The latter include conditioning: persistent alterations of synaptic transmission (long-term potentiation, LTP, and long-term depression, LTD) (Toyoda *et al.*, 2006).

Procedure and stimulation parameters

During TMS treatment, the patient is awake. A magnetic coil (figure-8 or round) is placed tangential to the skullcap (see Figure 7.2). In order to induce a magnetic field of about 2 T, a current of up to 10 000 A flows for 100–250 µs through the magnetic coil; this allows depolarization of the cortical neurons to a depth of 2–3 cm. The motor threshold is determined, so as to decide the intensity of the TMS stimulation

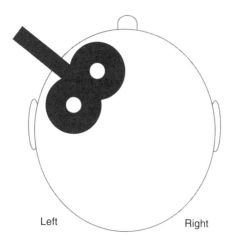

Left   Right

Figure 7.2   Figure-8 coil for repetitive transcranial magnetic stimulation at the region of the prefrontal dorsolateral cortex; that is, the position during depression treatment

(Di Lazzaro *et al.*, 2008). The frequency varies from 0.3 to 20.0 Hz (normally 5–20 Hz for TRD); stimulation and resting phases are intermittent. The treatment is applied daily for 2–3 weeks.

Side effects

rTMS is generally considered a safe treatment method. Side effects are transient headaches and induction of a seizure (<0.5%). There are several guidelines for the use of rTMS (Belmaker *et al.*, 2003; O'Reardon *et al.*, 2010; Wassermann, 1998).

Outlook

Theta-burst stimulation

During theta-burst stimulation (TBS), a series of impulses are delivered at high frequency, with a stimulus intensity of 80% of motor threshold. One study demonstrates efficacy (Paulus, 2005), but another restricts these results (Martin *et al.*, 2006).

Neuronavigation

One of the biggest sources of error in the application of TMS is imprecise coil position. With the recent development of neuro-navigation, it is now possible to adapt the coil position to an individual anatomical and functional image of the brain. This technique uses ultrasound and an infrared sensor for navigation.

Deep transcranial magnetic stimulation

The development of a magnetic coil for deep transcranial mag-netic stimulation (dTMS) makes stimulation of brain tissue possible up to depths of 8 cm below the scalp. An initial study has suggested an antidepressant effect (Rosenberg *et al.*, 2010).

Vagus nerve stimulation

The first therapeutic application of VNS in a patient with treatment-resistant epilepsy was carried out in 1988. In 2005, the FDA approved VNS for the treatment of therapy-resistant or recurrent uni- and bipolar depression. The requirement for the application of VNS was at least four different antidepressant treat-ments. In the EU, VNS is allowed for chronic or recurrent TRD or in patients unable or unwilling to tolerate pharmacotherapy.

Indications, contraindications and risk

In psychiatric indications, TRD is the main application for VNS (Bajbouj *et al.*, 2010; Schlaepfer *et al.*, 2008). Contraindications and risk include paralysis of the left vocal cord and cardiac and pulmonary diseases.

Mechanism of action

The mechanism of action is not completely elucidated. The vagus nerve is a complex structure with myelinated and nonmyelinated fibres. The afferent amount of fibre at the neck section is 80%, which conducts enteroceptive information from the periphery to the brain. Via the nucleus tractus solitaries, polysynaptic connections affect several cortical and subcortical areas, which play an important role in the regulation of affect (Kosel & Schlaepfer, 2002). This may be crucial to the progress of affective disorders (Nemeroff *et al.*, 2006). The vagal nerve has numerous projections, for example to the *locus coeruleus* and *raphe nuclei* (area of origin of the noradrenergic and serotonergic pathways); to the pontin and mesencephal nuclei; to the limbic structure (amygdala, hippocampus, thalamus and hypothalamus); and to cortical areas (prefrontal cortex) (Henry, 2002). Furthermore, changes in the concentration of monoamine (GABA, dopamine, serotonin and noradrenalin) (Ben-Menachem *et al.*, 1995) and normalization of corticotropin-releasing hormone (CRH)-induced adrenocorticotropin hormone (ACTH) secretion are associated with VNS. A US pilot study demonstrated a response of 30% after 10 weeks of VNS (Rush *et al.*, 2000), and even higher after 1 year (Nahas *et al.*, 2005), while a European study reported a response rate of 53% after 2 years (Bajbouj *et al.*, 2010; Schlaepfer *et al.*, 2008). Thus, VNS is not an acute treatment for depression. A previous effect following ECT seems to be a positive predictor for the efficacy of VNS (Sackheim *et al.*, 2007; Schlaepfer *et al.*, 2008).

Procedure and stimulation parameters

VNS is an invasive treatment, stimulating the left vagus nerve with two helicoidally electrodes at the cervical region. The electrodes are connected with an implanted generator (see

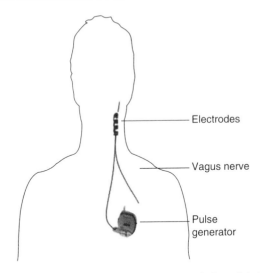

Figure 7.3   Vagus nerve stimulation (VNS). The helicoidal electrodes encompass the left vagus nerve and are connected with the implanted pulse generator

Figure 7.3). Typically, stimulation parameters are 0.25–3.5 mA, 20–30 Hz, 250–500 ms pulse width, 30-second duration of intermittent stimulation (on-time), followed by off-times of 3–5 minutes. The battery life, depending on stimulation parameters, varies between 8 and 12 years. It is important to note, that magnetic resonance imaging (MRI) of the head and neck can be performed with VNS (Cyberonics, 2008). Simultaneous application of VNS and ECT seems to be safe (Sharma *et al.*, 2009).

Side effects

There are differences between the side effects due to surgery and those due to stimulation. Operation-induced side effects are pain at the region of the scars, wound infections (≤3%)

and persistent paralysis of the left vocal cord (0.1%). Stimulation-induced side effects are asystole (0.1%), hoarseness and alterations of the voice (55%), cough (26%), pain (20%), respiratory problems (10%) and hypomania (1–3%).

Outlook

Transcutaneous vagus nerve stimulation

The tails of the vagus nerve proceed immediately along the skin surface at the region of the external meatus acusticus and can be stimulated by an electrode in transcutaneous vagus nerve stimulation (tVNS). Modulations in specific brain regions have been seen in imaging studies (Dietrich *et al.*, 2008), and changes in mood in a healthy group after tVNS treatment, but the efficacy is not clear for depressive disorders.

Deep-brain stimulation

DBS is a refined alternative to ablative neurosurgical interventions (Schlaepfer & Lieb, 2005). It was first implanted in psychiatric indications such as severe chronic TRD about 10 years ago. Globally, there are 140 patients with psychiatric diseases implanted with DBS, about 80 of whom suffer from TRD.

Indications, contraindications and risk

Indications for DBS are uni- and bipolar TRD, but its application is currently only possible in clinical studies. Contraindications are other axis II psychiatric disorders and risk concerning anaesthesia.

Mechanism of action and targets

The mechanism of action of DBS is mostly unknown. One hypothesis is that neuronal transmission induces chronic and high-frequency stimulation, which leads to inactivation of voltage-dependent neuronal ion channels. This mechanism leads to a functional lesion, analogous in efficacy to an ablative intervention. Modern functional, structural and molecular data have led to a new conceptualization of depression as a dysfunction of the networks that process motivational and affective stimuli (Krishnan & Nestler, 2010).

Previously published studies reported on case series of 10–20 patients (Table 7.1). The following target structures were the most investigated: nucleus accumbens (Figure 7.4), capsula interna and subgenual cingulate cortex (Brodman Areal, Cg25) (see Table 7.1). Furthermore, there are some case reports of DBS implantation in TRD at the inferior thalamus shaft (Jimenez et al., 2005), lateral habenula (Sartorius et al., 2010) and globus pallidus internus (Kosel et al., 2007). Some of the targets correspond through anatomical or functional conjunctions (neuronal networks), leading to overlapping effects in several areas of the brain. Published data show sustained antidepressant effects up to 6 years after DBS implantation in TRD patients (Kennedy et al., 2011), making it a promising treatment option.

Procedure and stimulation parameters

DBS is more invasive than the other brain-stimulation methods presented in this chapter. During a stereotactic operation, two thin electrodes are implanted in exactly defined areas of the brain. They are connected with a subclavicular or abdominal implanted generator. Typical parameters are constant stimulation at a frequency of 100 Hz, pulse width between 60 and 130 ms and voltage between 5 and 8 V.

Table 7.1 Target areas of deep-brain stimulation (DBS) of treatment-resistant depression (TRD). Response rates = 50% reduction of depression rating scales

Hypothesis	Target areas	Number of implanted patients	Response rate	References
Central structure of the reward system, anhedonia	Nucleus accumbens	13	1 year after implantation: 50%, with specially antianhedonic and anxiolytic effects	Bewernick, et al. (2010), Schlaepfer et al. (2008)
Theoretical explanation: historic lesion studies: efficacy of mood	Anterior capsula interna	17	6 months after implantation: 47%, last inquiry after average 37.4 months: 71%	Malone (2010), Malone et al. (2009)
Hyperactive through TRD	Subgenual cingular cortex (Brodman area, Cg25)	20	6 months after implantation: 60% 14 patients with 45% response after 2 years, 60% response after 3 years and 55% response at last follow-up visit up to 6 years	Lozano et al. (2008), Mayberg et al. (2005) Kennedy et al. (2011)

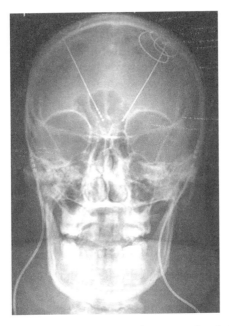

Figure 7.4 Bilateral deep-brain stimulation (DBS) of the nucleus accumbens. X-ray anterior–posterior of a treatment-resistant depression (TRD) patient in the Brain Stimulation Group at the University of Bonn

Side effects

There are differences between the side effects due to surgery and those due to stimulation. Operation-induced side effects are local infection (2–25%), intracranial haemorrhage (0.2–5.0%) and stroke and electrode damage. Stimulation-induced side effects are autonomic dysfunction, movement disorder, paraesthesia, dysarthria, diplopia, fear, agitation and hypomania.

Outlook

The results of the first uncontrolled studies of DBS are promising, and are consistent concerning the efficacy of DBS in various targets in TRD (Schlaepfer *et al.*, 2010). Two manufacturing companies (Medtronic and St Jude) have begun large pivotal studies of DBS in TRD of applicability to its wider use, and there are several smaller studies looking at new targets, such as the medial forebrain bundle (Coenen *et al.*, 2010).

Ethical considerations

There is some question over whether people suffering from TRD are restricted in their capacity to make rational decisions. Therefore, it is necessary to have an interdisciplinary evaluation of each individual case, with the participation of experienced psychiatrists, psychologists and neurosurgeons. Balanced and neutral information about DBS must be given to the patients and their relatives. A clear statement about the expected efficacy must be given. Crises in personal relationships and adaptive disorders independent of the effects of DBS need to be anticipated and counteracted by the treating experts (Synofzik & Schlapfer, 2008). It is also important that negative results be published. Thus, a central register of implanted patients in psychiatric disorders is of use (Schlaepfer & Fins, 2010).

Magnetic seizure therapy

MST is a further development of rTMS. In 1988, MST elicited first-time seizures in monkeys (Lisanby *et al.*, 2001a). The first induced MST seizure in humans occurred in 2000, at the University Hospital at Bern, Switzerland (Lisanby *et al.*, 2001b). The hypothesis was that MST induces a more focused generalized seizure, leading to less cognitive side effects as compared to ECT (Sackheim, 1994).

Indications, contraindications and risk

MST is only applied in clinical studies for uni- and bipolar TRD in four centres worldwide. Exclusion criteria are the risk of anaesthesia and metal parts in the head.

Mechanism of action

During MST, the brain areas involved in cognitive accomplishments are not affected (Lisanby, 2002), as they are during ECT (Rose et al., 2003). Patients undergoing MST are thus more rapidly reorientated than they would be following ECT (Kayser et al., 2011; Kirov et al., 2008). The exact mechanism of action is not fully understand, but there may be similar changes in neurotransmission and brain metabilism to those following ECT.

Procedure and stimulation parameters

A generalized seizure is elicited during intravenous anaesthesia, muscle relaxation and preoxygenation (much like in ECT). A magnetic field of up to 4T is needed to induce therapeutic seizures (Rowny et al., 2009). Thus, a special device is required for MST treatments. Usually, 10–12 MST treatments are administered in a series. The patient must wear earplugs against the clicking noise of the device. Common stimulation parameters are a frequency of 100Hz, amplitude of 100%, 100–800 pulses per train, stimulation duration of 1–8 seconds and repetition rate of up to 250pps. A twin coil is placed over the vertex (see Figure 7.5).

Side effects

The risk of serious side effects comes from the anaesthesia. Discomforts such as headache, nausea and cognitive disturbance,

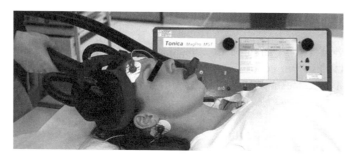

Figure 7.5 Magnetic seizure therapy (MST) at the University of Bonn, showing the prototype MagPro Magstim, with the twin coil placed on the vertex

which are common after ECT, do not occur with MST (Kayser *et al.*, 2009, 2011; Kirov *et al.*, 2008).

Outlook

Further studies are needed to reproduce the initial promising results. So far, 40 patients with TRD (26 at the University of Bonn) have shown equally good antidepressant results to those seen in ECT, but with less cognitive side effects.

References

Abrams, R. (2002) *Electroconvulsive Therapy*, Oxford University Press, New York, NY, USA.

American Psychiatric Association & Weiner, R. D. (2001) *The Practice of Electroconvulsive Therapy: Recommendations for Treatment, Training, and Privileging: A Task Force Report of the American Psychiatric Association*, American Psychiatric Association, Washington, DC, USA.

Baghai, T., Frey, R., Kasper, S. & Möller, H. (2004) *Elektrokonvulsionstherapie: Klinische und Wissenschaftliche Aspekte*, Springer, Vienna, Austria.

Bajbouj, M., Merkl, A., Schlaepfer, T. E. *et al.* (2010) Two-year outcome of vagus nerve stimulation in treatment-resistant depression. *J. Clin. Psychopharmacol.*, **30**(3), 273–281.

Barker, A. T., Jalinous, R. & Freeston, I. L. (1985) Non-invasive magnetic stimulation of human motor cortex. *Lancet*, **1**(8437), 1106–1107.

Bartholow, R. (1874) Experimental investigations into the functions of the human brain. *Am. J. Med. Sci.*, **67**, 305–313.

Belmaker, B., Fitzgerald, P., George, M. S. *et al.* (2003) Managing the risks of repetitive transcranial stimulation. *CNS Spectrum*, **8**(7), 489.

Ben-Menachem, E., Hamberger, A., Hedner, T. *et al.* (1995) Effects of vagus nerve stimulation on amino acids and other metabolites in the CSF of patients with partial seizures. *Epilepsy Res.*, **20**(3), 221–227.

Cerletti, U. & Bini, L. (1938) Un nuovo metodo di shockterapia: 'L'elettroshock'. *Boll. R. Accad. Med.*, **64**, 136–138.

Coenen, V. A., Schlaepfer, T. E., Maedler, B. & Panksepp, J. (2010) Cross-species affective functions of the medial forebrain bundle – implications for the treatment of affective pain and depression in humans. *Neurosci. Biobehav. Rev.*, **35**(9), 1971–1981.

Cyberonics (2008) Brief Summary of Safety Information for the VNS Therapy™ System. Epilepsy and Depression Indications.

Di Lazzaro, V., Ziemann, U. & Lemon, R. N. (2008) State of the art: physiology of transcranial motor cortex stimulation. *Brain Stim.: Basic Trans. Clin. Res. Neuromod.*, **1**(4), 345–362.

Dietrich, S., Smith, J., Scherzinger, C. *et al.* (2008) [A novel transcutaneous vagus nerve stimulation leads to brainstem and cerebral activations measured by functional MRI]. *Biomed. Tech. (Berlin)*, **53**(3), 104–111.

Fink, M. (2009) *Electroconvulsive Therapy: A Guide for Professionals and Their Patients*, Oxford University Press, New York, NY, USA.

George, M. S., Nahas, Z., Molloy, M. *et al.* (2000) A controlled trial of daily left prefrontal cortex TMS for treating depression. *Biol. Psychiatry*, **48**(10), 962–970.

Hayward, G., Mehta, M. A., Harmer, C. *et al.* (2007) Exploring the physiological effects of double-cone coil TMS over the medial frontal cortex on the anterior cingulate cortex: an H2(15)O PET study. *Eur. J. Neurosci.*, **25**(7), 2224–2233.

Henry, T. R. (2002) Therapeutic mechanisms of vagus nerve stimulation. *Neurology*, **59**(6 Suppl. 4), S3–14.

Herwig, U., Fallgatter, A. J., Hoppner, J. *et al.* (2007) Antidepressant effects of augmentative transcranial magnetic stimulation: randomised multicentre trial. *Brit. J. Psychiatry*, **191**, 441–448.

Hoffman, R. E. & Cavus, I. (2002) Slow transcranial magnetic stimulation, long-term depotentiation, and brain hyperexcitability disorders. *Am. J. Psychiatry*, **159**(7), 1093–1102.

Janicak, P. G., O'Reardon, J. P., Sampson, S. M. *et al.* (2008) Transcranial magnetic stimulation in the treatment of major depressive disorder: a comprehensive summary of safety experience from acute exposure, extended exposure, and during reintroduction treatment. *J. Clin. Psychiatry*, **69**(2), 222–232.

Janicak, P. G., Nahas, Z., Lisanby, S. H. *et al.* (2010) Durability of clinical benefit with transcranial magnetic stimulation (TMS) in the treatment of pharmacoresistant major depression: assessment of relapse during a 6-month, multisite, open-label study. *Brain Stimul.*, **3**(4), 187–199.

Jimenez, F., Velasco, F., Salin-Pascual, R. *et al.* (2005) A patient with a resistant major depression disorder treated with deep brain stimulation in the inferior thalamic peduncle. *Neurosurg.*, **57**(3), 585–593; discussion 593.

Kayser, S., Bewernick, B., Axmacher, N. & Schlaepfer, T. E. (2009) Magnetic seizure therapy of treatment-resistant depression in a patient with bipolar disorder. *J. ECT*, **25**(2), 137–140.

Kayser, S., Bewernick, B. H., Grubert, C. *et al.* (2011) Antidepressant effects, of magnetic seizure therapy and electroconvulsive therapy, in treatment-resistant depression. *J. Psychiatr. Res.*, **45**(5), 569–576.

Keck, M. E., Welt, T., Muller, M. B. *et al.* (2002) Repetitive transcranial magnetic stimulation increases the release of dopamine in the mesolimbic and mesostriatal system. *Neuropharmacol.*, **43**(1), 101–109.

Kennedy, S. H., Giacobbe, P., Rizvi, S. J. *et al.* (2011) Deep brain stimulation for treatment-resistant depression: follow-up after 3 to 6 years. *Am. J. Psychiatry*, **168**(5), 502–510.

Kirov, G., Ebmeier, K. P., Scott, A. I. *et al.* (2008) Quick recovery of orientation after magnetic seizure therapy for major depressive disorder. *Brit. J. Psychiatry*, **193**(2), 152–155.

Kosel, M. & Schlaepfer, T. E. (2002) Mechanisms and state of the art of vagus nerve stimulation. *J. ECT*, **18**(4), 189–192.

Kosel, M., Sturm, V., Frick, C. *et al.* (2007) Mood improvement after deep brain stimulation of the internal globus pallidus for tardive dyskinesia in a patient suffering from major depression. *J. Psychiatr. Res*, **41**(9), 801–803.

Krishnan, V. & Nestler, E. J. (2010) Linking molecules to mood: new insight into the biology of depression. *Am. J. Psychiatry*, **167**(11), 1305–1320.

Lisanby, S. H. (2002) Update on magnetic seizure therapy: a novel form of convulsive therapy. *J. ECT*, **18**(4), 182–188.

Lisanby, S. H. (2007) Electroconvulsive therapy for depression. *N. Engl. J. Med*, **357**(19), 1939–1945.

Lisanby, S. H., Luber, B., Finck, A. D. *et al.* (2001a) Deliberate seizure induction with repetitive transcranial magnetic stimulation in nonhuman primates. *Arch. Gen. Psychiatry*, **58**(2), 199–200.

Lisanby, S. H., Schlaepfer, T. E., Fisch, H. U. & Sackeim, H. A. (2001b) Magnetic seizure therapy of major depression. *Arch. Gen. Psychiatry*, **58**(3), 303–305.

Martin, P. G., Gandevia, S. C. & Taylor, J. L. (2006) Theta burst stimulation does not reliably depress all regions of the human motor cortex. *Clin. Neurophysiol.*, **117**(12), 2684–2690.

McCall, W. V., Reboussin, D. M., Weiner, R. D. & Sackeim, H. A. (2000) Titrated moderately suprathreshold vs fixed high-dose right unilateral electroconvulsive therapy: acute antidepressant and cognitive effects. *Arch. Gen. Psychiatry*, **57**(5), 438–444.

Mervaala, E., Kononen, M., Fohr, J. *et al.* (2001) SPECT and neuropsychological performance in severe depression treated with ECT. *J. Affect. Disord.*, **66**(1), 47–58.

Nahas, Z., Marangell, L. B., Husain, M. M. *et al.* (2005) Two-year outcome of vagus nerve stimulation (VNS) for treatment of major depressive episodes. *J. Clin. Psychiatry*, **66**(9), 1097–1104.

Nemeroff, C. B., Mayberg, H. S., Krahl, S. E. *et al.* (2006) VNS therapy in treatment-resistant depression: clinical evidence and putative neurobiological mechanisms. *Neuropsychopharmacol.*, **31**(7), 1345–1355.

Nobler, M. S., Oquendo, M. A., Kegeles, L. S. *et al.* (2001) Decreased regional brain metabolism after ect. *Am. J. Psychiatry*, **158**(2), 305–308.

O'Reardon, J. P., Solvason, H. B., Janicak, P. G. *et al.* (2007) Efficacy and safety of transcranial magnetic stimulation in the acute treatment of major depression: a multisite randomized controlled trial. *Biol. Psychiatry*, **62**(11), 1208–1216.

O'Reardon, J. P., Solvason, H. B., Janicak, P. G. *et al.* (2010) Reply regarding 'efficacy and safety of transcranial magnetic stimulation in the acute treatment of major depression: a multisite randomized controlled trial'. *Biol. Psychiatry*, **67**(2), e15–17.

Paulus, W. (2005) Toward establishing a therapeutic window for rTMS by theta burst stimulation. *Neuron*, **45**(2), 181–183.

Paus, T., Castro-Alamancos, M. A. & Petrides, M. (2001) Cortico-cortical connectivity of the human mid-dorsolateral frontal cortex and its modulation by repetitive transcranial magnetic stimulation. *Eur. J. Neurosci.*, **14**(8), 1405–1411.

Pfleiderer, B., Michael, N., Erfurth, A. *et al.* (2003) Effective electro-convulsive therapy reverses glutamate/glutamine deficit in the left anterior cingulum of unipolar depressed patients. *Psy. Res.*, **122**(3), 185–192.

Pogarell, O., Koch, W., Popperl, G. *et al.* (2007) Acute prefrontal rTMS increases striatal dopamine to a similar degree as D-amphetamine. *Psy. Res.*, **156**(3), 251–255.

Roepke, S., Luborzewski, A., Schindler, F. *et al.* (2011) Stimulus pulse-frequency-dependent efficacy and cognitive adverse effects of ultrabrief-pulse electroconvulsive therapy in patients with major depression. *J. ECT*, **27**(2), 109–113.

Rose, D., Fleischmann, P., Wykes, T. *et al.* (2003) Patients' perspectives on electroconvulsive therapy: systematic review. *BMJ*, **326**(7403), 1363.

Rosenberg, O., Shoenfeld, N., Zangen, A. *et al.* (2010) Deep TMS in a resistant major depressive disorder: a brief report. *Depression & Anxiety*, **27**(5), 465–469.

Rowny, S. B., Benzl, K. & Lisanby, S. H. (2009) Translational development strategy for magnetic seizure therapy. *Exp. Neurol.*, **219**(1), 27–35.

Rush, A. J., George, M. S., Sackeim, H. A. *et al.* (2000) Vagus nerve stimulation (VNS) for treatment-resistant depressions: a multi-center study. *Biol. Psychiatry*, **47**(4), 276–286.

Sackeim, H. A. (1994) Magnetic stimulation therapy and ECT. *Convuls. Ther.*, **10**, 255–258

Sackeim, H. A. (1999) The anticonvulsant hypothesis of the mechanisms of action of ECT: current status. *J. ECT*, **15**(1), 5–26.

Sackeim, H. A., Prudic, J., Devanand, D. P. *et al.* (1993) Effects of stimulus intensity and electrode placement on the efficacy and cognitive effects of electroconvulsive therapy. *N. Engl. J. Med.*, **328**(12), 839–846.

Sackeim, H. A., Prudic, J., Devanand, D. P. *et al.* (2000) A prospective, randomized, double-blind comparison of bilateral and right unilateral electroconvulsive therapy at different stimulus intensities. *Arch. Gen. Psychiatry*, **57**(5), 425–434.

Sackeim, H. A., Haskett, R. F., Mulsant, B. H. *et al.* (2001) Continuation pharmacotherapy in the prevention of relapse following electroconvulsive therapy: a randomized controlled trial. *JAMA*, **285**(10), 1299–1307.

Sackeim, H. A., Brannan, S. K., Rush, A. J. *et al.* (2007) Durability of antidepressant response to vagus nerve stimulation (VNS). *Int. J. Neuropsychopharmacol.*, **10**(6), 817–826.

Sartorius, A., Kiening, K. L., Kirsch, P. *et al.* (2010) Remission of major depression under deep brain stimulation of the lateral habenula in a therapy-refractory patient. *Biol. Psychiatry*, **67**(2), e9–11.

Schlaepfer, T. E. & Fins, J. J. (2010) Deep brain stimulation and the neuroethics of responsible publishing: when one is not enough. *JAMA*, **303**(8), 775–776.

Schlaepfer, T. E. & Lieb, K. (2005) Deep brain stimulation for treatment of refractory depression. *Lancet*, **366**(9495), 1420–1422.

Schlaepfer, T. E., Frick, C., Zobel, A. *et al.* (2008) Vagus nerve stimulation for depression: efficacy and safety in a European study. *Psychol. Med.*, **38**(5), 651–661.

Schlaepfer, T. E., George, M. S. & Mayberg, H. (2010) WFSBP guidelines on brain stimulation treatments in psychiatry. *World J. Biol. Psychiatry*, **11**(1), 2–18.

Scott, A. (2004) *The ECT Handbook*, 2nd edition, Royal College of Psychiatrists, London, UK.

Sharma, A., Chaturvedi, R., Sharma, A. & Sorrell, J. H. (2009) Electroconvulsive therapy in patients with vagus nerve stimulation. *J. ECT*, **25**(2), 141–143.

Siebner, H. R., Willoch, F., Peller, M. *et al.* (1998) Imaging brain activation induced by long trains of repetitive transcranial magnetic stimulation. *NeuroReport*, **9**(5), 943–948.

Siebner, H. R., Filipovic, S. R., Rowe, J. B. *et al.* (2003) Patients with focal arm dystonia have increased sensitivity to slow-frequency repetitive TMS of the dorsal premotor cortex. *Brain*, **126**(Pt 12), 2710–2725.

Spellman, T., Peterchev, A. V. & Lisanby, S. H. (2009) Focal electrically administered seizure therapy: a novel form of ECT illustrates the roles of current directionality, polarity, and electrode configuration in seizure induction. *Neuropsychopharmacol.*, **34**(8), 2002–2010.

Synofzik, M. & Schlaepfer, T. E. (2008) Stimulating personality: ethical criteria for deep brain stimulation in psychiatric patients and for enhancement purposes. *Biotechnol. J.*, **3**(12), 1511–1520.

Toyoda, H., Zhao, M. G. & Zhuo, M. (2006) NMDA receptor-dependent long-term depression in the anterior cingulate cortex. *Rev. Neurosci.*, **17**(4), 403–413.

UK ECT Review Group (2003) Efficacy and safety of electroconvulsive therapy in depressive disorders: a systematic review and meta-analysis. *Lancet*, **361**, 799–808.

Wahlund, B. & von Rosen, D. (2003) ECT of major depressed patients in relation to biological and clinical variables: a brief overview. *Neuropsychopharmacol.*, **28**(Suppl. 1), S21–26.

Wassermann, E. M. (1998) Risk and safety of repetitive transcranial magnetic stimulation: report and suggested guidelines from the International Workshop on the Safety of Repetitive Transcranial Magnetic Stimulation, June 5–7, 1996. *Electroencephalogr. Clin. Neurophysiol.*, **108**(1), 1–16.

Young, E. A., Spencer, R. L. & McEwen, B. S. (1990) Changes at multiple levels of the hypothalamo-pituitary adrenal axis following repeated electrically induced seizures. *Psychoneuroendocrinol.*, **15**(3), 165–172.

Ziemann, U., Paulus, W., Nitsche, M. A. *et al.* (2008) Consensus: motor cortex plasticity protocols. *Brain Stim.: Basic Trans. Clin. Res. Neuromod.*, **1**(3), 164–182.

CHAPTER 8

The Role of Psychotherapy in the Management of Treatment-resistant Depression

Michael E. Thase

*Perelman School of Medicine, University of Pennsylvania,
Philadelphia Veterans Affairs Medical Center, PA, USA;
University of Pittsburgh Medical Center, PA, USA*

Summary

Although treatment-resistant depression (TRD) is often approached from a psychopharmacological perspective, unremitting depressions that do not respond to conventional antidepressant strategies develop within intra- and interpersonal contexts that provide targets for psychotherapeutic interventions. Thus, just as time-limited psychotherapies such as cognitive behavioural therapy (CBT) and interpersonal psychotherapy (IPT) have emerged as empirically supported alternatives to pharmacotherapy for uncomplicated depressions, so too are a

Treatment-resistant Depression, First Edition. Edited by Siegfried Kasper
and Stuart Montgomery.
© 2013 John Wiley & Sons, Ltd. Published 2013 by John Wiley & Sons, Ltd.

number of psychotherapies being adapted for and tested in TRD. This chapter outlines the rationale for using psychotherapy in patients who have not responded to antidepressants, provides an overview of some of the issues complicating research in this area and reviews the results from relevant controlled studies. Finally, some of the common or 'core' principles of psychotherapy for patients with difficult-to-treat depressive episodes are summarized.

Introduction

This chapter examines the role of psychotherapy in the management of adults suffering from TRD. It begins with a brief discussion of the natural history of depression and considers the relative importance of specific and nonspecific factors in the response to various forms of treatment. It is suggested that, given the relatively modest size of specific drug effects in contemporary randomized controlled trials (RCTs), it should not be surprising that some people who do not respond to one or more adequate trials of antidepressants can still be good candidates for psychotherapy, particularly when these modalities target different aspects of a very heterogeneous illness. The relevant literature is reviewed pertaining to the effectiveness of several forms of psychotherapy in studies of major depressive disorder (MDD), then a more in-depth review of the several studies of psychotherapy that have focused on patients with TRD is presented. Although the literature on this latter topic is far from definite, there is evidence that patients who have not responded to one or two trials of antidepressant medication have a 30–50% chance of responding to a focused psychotherapy, which approximates the likelihood of benefit that can be expected with most pharmacological alternatives. Finally, indications for psychotherapy in TRD are suggested and some general therapeutic principles that transcend specific theoretical models are summarized.

Natural history of depression

Depression is usually characterized by an episodic course: most people will recover from an index depressive episode, whether or not they receive treatment, within 1 or 2 years. However, about 20% of untreated depressive episodes become chronic (i.e. persist for longer than 2 years), and there is a 'renewed' risk of chronicity with each depressive episode. Thus, although depression can still be thought of as an illness with a relatively good prognosis, especially when compared to conditions such as schizophrenia or bipolar affective disorder, a significant minority of people who become depressed will develop persistent, unremitting and potentially life-ruining illnesses.

As most people who develop chronic depressive disorders have never had a single adequate trial of a proven therapy, prompt and vigorous treatment is postulated to be the most reliable way of preventing chronicity. The most common form of MDD, namely a relatively acute, nonpsychotic episode of mild to moderate symptom severity, is responsive to a remarkably diverse group of interventions, ranging from – on the less intensive end of a continuum of treatment invasiveness – watchful waiting, brief supportive counselling and aerobic exercise to – at the more intensive end – complex multidrug regimens and neuromodulation strategies such as repetitive transcranial magnetic stimulation (rTMS) and electroconvulsive therapy (ECT). The psychotherapies that have been empirically validated as effective treatments of MDD would generally be classified as falling on the left side of such a treatment continuum, perhaps immediately adjacent to some of the safer, newer-generation antidepressant medications. The diversity of therapies that are used to treat depression underscores the clinical heterogeneity of MDD.

For most people seeking treatment for depression in the first decades of the 21st century, antidepressant medications and psychotherapy – either singly or in combination – are considered the first line of therapy. In practice, many people who have a strong preference for psychotherapy 'vote with their feet' by initially consulting a nonmedical behavioural health provider, such as a psychologist, social worker or licensed counsellor. Such a depressed person might not even consider treatment with an antidepressant until months or even years have been spent in psychotherapy. Others, by contrast, first consult their primary care provider and begin treatment with antidepressant pharmacotherapy. Some of these medication-treated depressed patients have no interest in seeing a counsellor or psychotherapist, but others do not know that psychotherapy is a viable option.

There has been a strong temporal trend in the USA over the past several decades pertaining to the use of first-line treatments for MDD: the number of depressed patients receiving psychotherapy or counselling has decreased and the use of antidepressant medication has increased (Olfson *et al.*, 2002). With respect to types of medication, the term 'antidepressant pharmacotherapy' has become almost synonymous with the selective serotonin reuptake inhibitors (SSRIs) and serotonin norepinephrine reuptake inhibitors (SNRIs), which currently account for over 80% of all antidepressant prescriptions. The changing patterns of use of treatments of depression in part reflect the shift in treatment to primary care settings, where antidepressant pharmacotherapy can be delivered with less professional contact and at a lower cost than psychotherapy. Specifically, both the SSRIs and the SNRIs are now available in generic formulations and, over the course of 6 or 8 weeks (i.e. an adequate duration for a course of pharmacotherapy), the provider may schedule only two or three follow-up visits.

Despite what appears to be a quite favourable value proposition, there are growing concerns that antidepressants are being overprescribed and that their benefits have been overvalued. For example, although it has long been taught that antidepressants have a 67% response rate in MDD, more careful inspection of RCT datasets indicates that only about 50% of those who begin therapy will actually benefit, with only about two-thirds of responders remitting by the end of the eighth week of therapy

(Thase, 2011). There are also legitimate concerns about the generalizability of RCT populations. In the Sequenced Treatment Alternatives to Relieve Depression (STAR*D) study, for example, fewer than one-quarter of adults seeking treatment for MDD met standard RCT inclusion criteria, and these patients were significantly more likely to remit during a prospective treatment trial with the SSRI citalopram (Wisniewski *et al.*, 2009). Among those who likely would have been excluded from an RCT, only 39% had responded and fewer than 25% had remitted by the end of up to 14 weeks of therapy with citalopram ≤60 mg/day. Thus, one can be fairly confident that – in the 'real world' – an initial course of antidepressant medication will fail to produce the desired benefit one-half of the time.

Among those who do benefit, recent research suggests that the so-called specific effects of treatment (i.e. the pharmacological actions of the drug) are dwarfed by the nonspecific or 'placebo' effects, which include the therapeutic effects of being cared for, the passage of time and repeated assessment (Thase, 2011). In fact, metaanalyses of RCTs of newer-generation antidepressants suggest that the specific effects of treatment are relatively small, with effect sizes on the order of 0.3–0.4 (see, for example, Kirsch *et al.*, 2008; Thase *et al.*, 2011; Turner *et al.*, 2008). With respect to response rates, the nonspecific elements of treatment account for up to 70% of the benefit of pharmacotherapy in the modern era (i.e. 35% divided by 50%), with a number needed to treat (NNT) for specific benefit typically ranging between 5 and 10 (Thase, 2011). Thus, among a hypothetical group of 10 people seeking treatment for depression, at least 5 will not respond and perhaps only 1 or 2 will actually respond because of the specific pharmacological actions of an antidepressant.

There are no reliable means available to help clinicians identify those who are likely to respond to a placebo or, conversely, to identify those depressed patients whose recovery might hinge on receiving an active medication. It is generally true that, in placebo-controlled RCTs, placebo response rates are higher among depressed patients with more acute, milder and relatively uncomplicated illnesses, and the likelihood of placebo response is lower for those with more severe, chronic or complex illnesses (Thase *et al.*, 2001). Similar findings are observed in longitudinal studies: patients who develop more chronic, unremitting depressions tend to have more severe, comorbid (both psychiatric and medical conditions) and otherwise complicated disorders (Corey-Lisle *et al.*, 2004; Sherbourne *et al.*, 2004; Souery *et al.*, 2007). Some of the complicating effects associated with chronicity or nonresponse to antidepressant therapies include socioeconomic factors, such as poverty and unemployment, and interpersonal factors, such as low social support and marital discord (Fava & Visani, 2008; Rubenstein *et al.*, 2007; Thase & Howland, 1994). In general terms, the higher the number of indicators of treatment difficulty in the past, the greater the likelihood of developing TRD going forward (Souery *et al.*, 2007). Thus, although the constructs of chronicity and treatment resistance are not synonymous, there are a number of shared risks, and once established, neither condition is likely to spontaneously remit (Thase *et al.*, 2001).

One important component of the nonspecific benefit of treatment is the strength of the helping alliance. Although more often discussed with respect to psychotherapy, the helping alliance likely facilitates most, if not all, forms of treatment. In one RCT, a strong therapeutic alliance was as predictive for pharmacotherapy response – in this case both imipramine and placebo – as for response to formal psychotherapies (in this case, cognitive behavioural therapy (CBT) and interpersonal psychotherapy (IPT)) (Krupnick *et al.*, 1996).

The value of a strong therapeutic alliance no doubt reflects at least in part the depressed person's capacity to work productively and collaboratively in a dyadic relationship with the helping professional. It is also likely true that a strong alliance reflects the helping professional's skill and ability to engage the depressed person in the ongoing and iterative process of treatment, which can be a considerable advantage when progress is slow and revisions must be made to the treatment plan.

Pessimism and demoralization, which are prototypic cognitive symptoms of depression, are exacerbated by failure experiences and are common features of people with TRD (Thase *et al.*, 2001). Indeed, pessimism and demoralization can derail the therapeutic process, and as observed in STAR*D, each unsuccessful course of therapy will result in some number of people withdrawin from treatment (Rush *et al.*, 2006).

A somewhat related psychosocial determinant of nonresponse is nonadherence (Thase *et al.*, 2001). Some people remain in treatment but do not take their medications in the way that they have been prescribed. Medications that are either not taken or taken haphazardly do not exert the expected benefits and nonadherence to pharmacotherapy is an oft underestimated determinant of poor outcomes (Mitchell, 2006). It therefore behoves clinicians to try to ensure that a medication has actually been taken in an adequate dose and duration before assuming that it has 'failed' to deliver the hoped-for benefit.

In summary, depressed people who have not responded to one or more courses of antidepressant therapy have not obtained the hoped-for clinically meaningful benefits from either the specific or the nonspecific elements of treatment. They are, in turn, unlikely to remit spontaneously and less likely to respond to subsequent courses of therapy than treatment-naïve individuals.

As there have been no longitudinal placebo-controlled studies of multistep treatment regimens, it is difficult to gauge to what extent the decrement in antidepressant response is attributable to a dissipation of nonspecific effects versus an actual loss of antidepressant efficacy. Nevertheless, in RCTs using an enrichment strategy known as the sequential parallel group design (see Fava *et al.*, 2003), in which it is possible to be re-randomized to a second course of placebo therapy, it can be shown that the placebo response can diminish while the magnitude of the drug-versus-placebo difference increases. Thus, there is reason for cautious therapeutic optimism even when it is clear that the patient is suffering from a more difficult-to-treat depressive disorder.

Depression-focused psychotherapy

Emerging in the 1960s and 1970s in response to concerns about the use of longer-term, psychodynamically focused psychotherapy for the treatment of depression, several models of 'depression-focused psychotherapy' are now considered to be viable alternatives to pharmacotherapy. The most fully developed and best studied psychotherapies include Beck's cognitive therapy (CT) (Beck *et al.*, 1979) and IPT (Klerman *et al.*, 1984), although a broader array of conceptually related interventions referred to as CBT also show merit. These therapies share several common elements: (1) they are time-limited (typically 8–16 weeks in duration); (2) they focus primarily on the here and now, rather than the past; (3) the aim to treat the depressive episode as the primary goal; and (4) they follow a specified procedure and use a set of techniques guided by a particular theory of depression or behaviour change. These interventions are further differentiated from more traditional psychodynamic psychotherapies by the fact that, at the time of their introduction, their utility for treatment of depression was established by RCTs. In this way, advocates of the depression-focused psychotherapies shared the empirical zeitgeist that was being championed by biologically orientated researchers. Although advocates of psychoanalytic psychotherapy once rejected the ability of RCTs to empirically validate the utility of their clinical methods, over the past several decades a literature pertaining to the use of psychodynamic psychotherapy for the treatment of depression has begun to emerge (see, for example, Driessen *et al.*, 2010a).

Evidence that psychotherapy is as effective as pharmacotherapy

Although psychotherapy is the leading alternative to pharmacotherapy for first-line treatment of MDD, the levels of empirical support for these modalities are not comparable. In contrast to antidepressants, for which a series of large and reasonably well-controlled RCTs is required by regulatory authorities such as the US Food and Drug Administration (FDA) before they can be approved for general use, there are few regulatory bodies overseeing the merits of various psychotherapies and essentially no commercial entities that underwrite the research necessary to develop, pilot test, refine and confirm the benefits of new models. As a result, there have always been – and in all likelihood always will be – many more studies of antidepressant medications than of depression-focused psychotherapies. Beyond the lack of funding, there are also conceptual and methodological issues that make it harder to conduct well-controlled studies of psychotherapy. For example, whereas a pill placebo is a perfect control for an RCT of a novel medication, no such ideal exists for studies of novel psychotherapies. Waiting-list control groups are often used early in treatment development, but this condition does not convey the essential components to control for nonspecific benefits. In fact, a waiting-list control group, which only accounts for the impact of the passage of time and repeated assessment, might inadvertently convey the expectation that patients should 'wait for something better'.

When a novel psychotherapy appears to have a meaningful benefit, it is usually compared to either a 'pseudotherapy' or an established treatment, such as an antidepressant medication. With respect to active comparators, many of the early studies on focused psychotherapies were conducted before the concept of statistical power was fully appreciated and long before the notion of therapeutic equivalence, as tested using the so-called 'noninferiority design', was accepted. Looking back, none of the first- or second-generation comparative studies were large enough to afford the statistical power needed to conduct an actual test of noninferiority; such studies require 200–300 patients per arm (Thase, 2011).

With respect to 'pseudotherapies', some effort has been directed at developing the equivalent of a placebo psychotherapy, which would convey the elements of contact, support and alliance without specific, theoretically guided interventions.

It has been shown that the magnitude of the effect of a 'pseudotherapy' is largely determined by the allegiance of the investigative team, and if the intervention is known to be a 'dud', it does not provide a very strong control condition (Gaffan *et al.*, 1996). The metaanalysis by Cuijpers *et al.* (2012) suggests that nondirective psychotherapy, if administered and delivered by 'true believers' to minimize allegiance bias, constitutes a very strong control group, such that the magnitudes of the 'specific effects' of focused psychotherapies are probably comparable to those of pharmacotherapy. What is still not known is the extent to which specific effects of psychotherapy and pharmacotherapy overlap.

Despite these limitations, real progress has been made over the past 40 years and a number of comparative studies of time-limited cognitive, behavioural, interpersonal and – more recently – psychodynamic psychotherapies have been completed. As is the case in the pharmacotherapy literature, there are inconsistencies in results across studies. Nevertheless, the results of metaanalyses and systematic reviews indicate that these focused interventions are indeed efficacious when compared to waiting-list or minimal-contact control conditions across 8–16 weeks of treatment, with a magnitude of improvement and likelihood of response/remission that are generally comparable to antidepressant pharmacotherapy (Cuijpers *et al.*, 2010, 2011; Driessen *et al.*, 2010a; Hollon *et al.*, 2005; Parikh *et al.*, 2009). Moreover, although the results of a secondary analysis from one relatively large comparative study suggest that the tricyclic antidepressant (TCA) imipramine may be more effective than CT in outpatients with more severe depression (Elkin *et al.*, 1995), the findings of other studies (DeRubeis *et al.*, 2005, 2006) and metaanalyses (DeRubeis *et al.*, 1999; Driessen *et al.*, 2010b) suggest that severity *per se* does not define an upward boundary to psychotherapy efficacy, at least with respect to treating nonpsychotic outpatients with MDD.

There is also growing evidence from comparative studies to suggest that cognitive, behavioural, interpersonal and time-limited psychodynamic forms of therapy have relatively comparable efficacies in studies of depressed outpatients (Jakobsen *et al.*, 2012a; Thoma *et al.*, 2012). Among these therapies, the only clearly distinguishing factor may be that there is more evidence that CT has a relatively 'durable' benefit (i.e. patients are less likely to relapse after cessation of therapy than those withdrawn from antidepressants) (Vittengl *et al.*, 2007). However, even in this case it must be noted that superior longer-term outcomes for CT have not been observed in studies that compare CT to other credible psychotherapies, such as IPT (Shea *et al.*, 1991) or behavioural activation (Dobson *et al.*, 2008).

There is also a growing consensus on the merits of and indications for combining psychotherapy and pharmacotherapy. In a metaanalysis using individual patient data drawn from a series of studies conducted at the University of Pittsburgh Medical Center, combined treatment was found to be superior to psychotherapy alone, with a marginal overall advantage in remission rates of about 10% among milder patients and a much larger advantage (~40%) among patients with more severe recurrent depression (Thase *et al.*, 1996). The advantage of combined treatment over pharmacotherapy alone has also been confirmed by metaanalyses of RCTs (Cuijpers *et al.*, 2009; Jakobsen *et al.*, 2012b; Pampallona *et al.*, 2004). The evidence of an advantage is less consistent, however, when combined treatment is compared to a well-crafted psychotherapy (de Maat *et al.*, 2007). Severe recurrent depression (Thase *et al.*, 1996) and chronic depression (Keller *et al.*, 2000) may represent the strongest indications for combined therapy instead of psychotherapy alone.

As the evidence that focused forms of psychotherapy are effective alternatives to antidepressants has increased, so too have concerns about the availability of these therapies to the general public. It is likely that, even today, only a minority of therapists practising outside of research studies actually provide a form of psychotherapy that could be readily identified as CT or IPT, or one of the other focused psychotherapies. Although one can be somewhat optimistic that the findings of research studies generalize at least to some extent to community practice, little is known about the effectiveness of 'eclectic' psychotherapy in 'real-world' settings.

Studies of TRD

As reviewed elsewhere in more detail (Thase & Howland, 1994; Thase *et al.*, 2001), until the last few years only relatively small 'pilot' studies had been conducted in TRD; collectively, the results of these studies suggested that some patients with even relatively advanced forms of TRD could benefit from focused psychotherapy. Despite such promise, however, the lack of evidence from well-controlled and adequately powered studies tended to stymie attempts to integrate these modalities into evidence-based algorithms for TRD (see, for example, Gaynes *et al.*, 2011; Stimpson *et al.*, 2002; Trivedi *et al.*, 2009).

One of the overarching goals of STAR*D was to conduct the first such study (Rush *et al.*, 2004). Specifically, Beck's model of CT was included in STAR*D Level 2, as one of the options to be compared among patients who did not remit with an adequate trial of citalopram. The randomized design used in STAR*D included comparisons of CT as both a switch (i.e. instead of an alternative antidepressant medication) and an adjunct to ongoing citalopram therapy (in comparison to two adjunctive medication strategies) (Thase *et al.*, 2007). Unfortunately, an unforeseen consequence of the use of the special randomization procedure, which enabled the patient–physician dyads to 'cross off' certain options, was that only 102 of the planned 400 patients were randomized to the CT arms, which greatly limited the statistical power of the planned comparisons.

Although the unexpectedly high incidence of patients opting out of randomization strata that included CT might be interpreted as an indication that psychotherapy is not a desirable treatment option for TRD patients who have not responded to antidepressants, there are several reasons to believe that this is not the correct interpretation of the finding. For example, the very same problem with equipoise stratified randomization similarly prevented the planned comparisons of the adjunctive and switching-medication strategies (Wisniewski *et al.*, 2007), yet no one has suggested that this indicates one or the other of these strategies is not acceptable to patients in 'real-world' settings. Moreover, other studies utilizing crossover designs (Schatzberg *et al.*, 2005) or fewer comparison groups (Kocsis *et al.*, 2009b; Wiles *et al.*, 2012) have had no difficulty getting people who have not responded to antidepressants to agree to receive psychotherapy. Thus, rather than specifically singling out psychotherapy as a less acceptable option, it appears that STAR*D patients exercised the choice afforded by the design to narrow the number of possible treatments available for random assignment.

In any event, the STAR*D patients who were randomized to CT generally fared as well as those who were randomized to alternative medication strategies (Thase *et al.*, 2007). As a switch option, the CBT group had comparable outcomes and significantly fewer side effects than the group that was switched from citalopram to an alternative antidepressant (sertraline, bupropion or venlafaxine ER). As an adjunct strategy, the CBT and pharmacotherapy groups showed comparable outcomes and tolerabilities, although the group that received adjunctive pharmacotherapy (either buspirone or bupropion added to citalopram) had a significantly more rapid onset of benefit. Specifically, patients who received adjunctive pharmacotherapy remitted several weeks faster than those who received adjunctive CBT.

More recently, a study known by the acronym CoBalT examined the effectiveness of adding CT to ongoing antidepressant therapy in primary care settings in the UK (Wiles *et al.*, 2012). In this study, patients who scored at least 14 on the Beck Depression Inventory (BDI) despite at least 6 weeks of antidepressant pharmacotherapy were recruited from 73 UK general practices. Only about 18% of the patients judged to be eligible to participate declined randomization. Although the study entry criteria were inclusive for mild depression, the mean BDI score for the randomized sample (n = 469) was 31.8, which is indicative of a relatively persistent moderate-to-severe level of depression despite ongoing pharmacotherapy. Patients were randomized to either usual care alone (n = 235) or in combination with CT (n = 234). The therapy protocol permitted up to 18 sessions of individual CT within the first 6 months post-randomization. The outcomes of interest were assessed periodically across 1 year, including at 6 months (i.e. the end of acute-phase therapy) and 12 months (i.e. at least 6 months after the end of therapy). The study had good retention of participants: 422 (90%) were followed up at 6 months and 396 (84%) were evaluated at 12 months post-randomization. The group that received adjunctive CT showed significant effects on most measures, including a highly significant difference in the primary outcome, response rates (as defined by a 50% reduction in BDI scores) at month 6 (modified intent-to-treat rates: 46.1 versus 21.6%; NNT = 5). A smaller but still clinically meaningful difference was also observed in remission rates at month 6 (27.7 versus 15.0%; NNT = 7). Significant differences favouring the group that received adjunctive CT were seen at the 12-month follow-up on most measures. Thus, in contrast to STAR*D, the findings of the CoBalT study indicate that adjunctive CT is both a very acceptable option and provides a large and clinically meaningful benefit.

Several larger-scale studies of chronic depression are also relevant to the question of the merits of psychotherapy for antidepressant nonresponders. In the first, which was a second phase of the large study of Keller et al. (2000), patients who had not responded to 12 weeks of therapy with either nefazodone or a variant of CBT known as the Cognitive Behavioral Analysis System of Psychotherapy (CBASP), had the opportunity to switch modalities to receive 12 weeks of additional treatment with the alternative modality (Schatzberg et al., 2005). The partial crossover design of this study does not permit valid comparisons of the two modalities. Nevertheless, the patients who received CBASP after first not responding to nefazodone were more likely to complete the second course of treatment than the group that was switched from CBASP to nefazodone (53/61 (87%) versus 57/79 (72%)) and had a higher intention to treat (ITT) response rate (57 versus 42%). Indeed, comparing across studies, while there appeared to be a decrement in the response rate among the two groups treated with nefazodone, CBASP was as likely to work in the second-step position as it was as a first-line therapy.

A second trial of chronic depression used a prospective, randomized design to compare CBASP and supportive psychotherapy among patients who had first not responded to an adequate course of pharmacotherapy. This study, known by the acronym REVAMP (Kocsis et al., 2009a), used more commonly prescribed first- and second-line antidepressants (instead of nefazodone) and, like STAR*D, employed relatively few exclusion criteria. A total of 491 chronically depressed patients who did not respond to an initial course of antidepressant medication were randomized to one of three options: switching to a second course of antidepressant medication, switching to CBASP in addition to a second course of antidepressant medication and switching to brief supportive psychotherapy in addition to a second course of antidepressant medication. Despite having adequate statistical power to detect relatively modest between-group differences, there was no evidence that the addition of psychotherapy – whether specific or simply supportive – improved outcomes as compared to simply changing antidepressant therapies. None of the three groups actually fared particularly well, however, with ITT response rates of about 40%. One possible explanation for this disappointing finding is that the duration of therapy – 12 weeks – was simply not long enough to detect an additive benefit in such a chronically ill group of antidepressant nonresponders.

If CBASP is not the best alternative to CT, it may be that other psychotherapies that have not yet been studied systematically in TRD hold more promise. It is also possible that particular forms of psychotherapy may be good matches for some TRD patients and not for others. For example, in one comparative trial of MDD, patients with high levels of dysfunctional thoughts, poor social functioning and limited social supports did particularly poorly with CT but responded reasonably well to a simpler behavioural-activation intervention (Coffman *et al.*, 2007). Other groups have advocated adapting mindfulness-based cognitive therapy (MCBT) (Eisendrath *et al.*, 2011) and dialectical behaviour therapy (DBT) (Harley *et al.*, 2008) for work with patients with more advanced forms of TRD. As the most difficult patients may warrant longer courses of psychotherapy, one must also reconsider the potential role of more traditional psychodynamic psychotherapies (Luten & Blatt, 2012). Indeed, several proof-of-concept studies of this approach are currently underway (Roose, 2012; Taylor *et al.*, 2012).

Assessing patients for psychotherapy

In current practice, the focused psychotherapies are indicated for the outpatient treatment of nonpsychotic forms of MDD, either as a single modality or in combination with ongoing pharmacotherapy. If one is following an algorithm in which two courses of antidepressant pharmacotherapy are required before using the term 'TRD', a depression-focused psychotherapy will be thought of at the same time as a TCA or adjunctive therapy with lithium salts, thyroid hormone or a second-generation antipsychotic (SGA). Although ECT might also be considered for treatment of patients with this level of treatment resistance, most clinicians will not be weighing the relative merits of psychotherapy versus this very intensive modality. One will likewise think of adjunctive therapy with an SGA ahead of psychotherapy for the subset of patients with psychotic features or severe melancholia. Conversely, one might think of switching to a monoamine oxidase inhibitor (MAOI) for a TRD patient with marked reverse-neurovegetative features. Yet, for the majority of patients not responding to antidepressants, who are characterized as having nonpsychotic, nonmelancholic depressive symptoms, the clinical evidence on differential therapeutics becomes quite sparse. For such patients, preference and feasibility are perhaps the most important factors: would the patient like to give psychotherapy a try and is there a capable therapist available?

Identifying goals for therapy

Many patients with TRD feel overwhelmed by their current circumstances and have difficulty focusing on specific problems. In such cases, it can be useful to collaboratively develop a problem list at the outset of therapy. One almost universal problem area in TRD is decreased interest in pleasurable or rewarding activities. Helping patients to reengage in the enjoyable activities that helped to make their lives worth living can therefore have a mood-lifting effect. In CBT, this is explicitly done early in therapy by using a schedule of daily activities; typically, patients are asked to record not only what they are doing, but also how they are feeling, and to grade the extent to which the planned activity is associated with feelings of pleasure and mastery. In this way, the daily activity schedule becomes an important source of information about how the depressed person is spending his or her time and what activities are associated with feeling better or worse.

The problem list may also include particularly troublesome symptoms of the unremitting depressive syndrome. Some of the more commonly observed persistent symptoms are fatigue, poor concentration, anxiety and insomnia. With growing recognition of the values of measurement-based care, ongoing use of a validated self-report scale can provide not only a more comprehensive assessment of a patient's level of severity but also a reliable method by which to monitor treatment outcomes. Other assessments, such as a measure of dysfunctional attitudes or completion of an inventory of interpersonal problems, may be used in particular forms of psychotherapy to clarify potential targets for treatment.

Regardless of the type of psychotherapy utilized, it is helpful from the outset for the therapist to convey an attitude of 'cautious optimism' and, if appropriate, share examples of successful treatment of similar patients. Ideally, the therapist can also describe how aspects of the therapy can be adapted to address the patient's most important or troublesome problems.

Another example of psychoeducation might be to provide a description of how TRD differs from other forms of depression from the perspective of the particular theoretical model of psychotherapy that will be utilized. In my own practice, I find it helpful to describe an illness model that incorporates both medical and psychosocial factors and a model of treatment that draws heavily on the concept of rehabilitation. Although it is true that TRD is not analogous to diabetes or stroke, most patients do know someone with a chronic health problem who has benefited from some form of rehabilitative therapy. When appropriate for the educational level and interests of the patient, I may also use examples of research involving positron emission tomography (PET) or functional magnetic resonance imaging (fMRI) scans to illustrate how psychotherapy, as compared to pharmacotherapy, can target regions of the brain that are of relevance to persistent depressive states (see, for example, Goldapple *et al.*, 2004; Kennedy *et al.*, 2007).

Box 8.1 summarizes some of the general or transtheoretical principles of psychotherapy with patients suffering from TRD. These include the following: (1) therapy will be active and will involve more than simple discussion of 'issues'; (2) the impact of therapy on depressive symptoms will be monitored and success will be measured, at least in part, by symptom reduction; (3) although the therapeutic relationship is not the primary 'vehicle' for therapeutic change, a strong collaborative alliance will enhance the chances of a successful outcome, and as such, apparent strains in the therapeutic alliance will be addressed whenever possible; (4) benefit is more likely to occur through a series of small steps than dramatic sudden gains; (5) the impact

Box 8.1   Suggested guidelines for psychotherapy with a patient suffering from treatment-resistant depression (TRD). Adapted from Thase & Howland (1994) and Thase *et al.* (2001)

- Try to emphasize a collaborative therapeutic relationship and identify both measurable, stepwise, short-term goals and more aspirational, longer-term goals.
- Set cautiously optimistic expectations for benefit. Provide examples of successful treatment of others with similar problems.
- Keep track of the levels of depressive symptoms and monitor outcomes over time.
- Provide psychoeducation about depression and its treatment and draw upon the medical model of rehabilitation as an example of minimizing the impact of 'bone fide' illnesses.
- Take an active role, leaning more toward coaching than reflective listening.
- Involve the patient's spouse or significant other whenever possible.
- Use specific therapeutic strategies to address relevant symptoms (e.g. relaxation training, activity scheduling, problem solving, cognitive restructuring).
- Meet as often as possible and, if necessary, shorten sessions to enhance learning and retention.
- Be mindful of rifts in and potential ruptures of the therapeutic alliance and don't be bashful about addressing them proactively. Obtain feedback about the patient's perceptions of progress and areas of difficulties.
- Don't be afraid to change therapeutic directions if the original plan is not leading to results.
- Use homework assignments and in-session rehearsal to facilitate development of new coping skills.

Adapted from Thase & Howland (1994) and Thase, Friedman and Howland (2001).

of specific interventions will be assessed and interventions that are not helping will be revised or replaced iteratively until benefit is obtained; and (6) although therapy is time-limited and not indefinite, the 'dose' – in terms of both session frequency and overall duration – will be titrated to meet the needs of the individual patient.

Conclusions

The depression-focused psychotherapies are pragmatic and potentially personally relevant approaches that comprise the primary nonpharmacological alternative for outpatients who have not responded to first- and second-line antidepressant medications. Although the results of studies such as STAR*D and REVAMP provide sobering evidence of the limitations of these approaches, the more strikingly positive results of the CoBalT study are grounds for therapeutic optimism: the depression-focused therapies are likely to offer as much chance of benefit as any alternative pharmacological approach that might be considered for a patient who has not responded to antidepressant therapy, with a more favourable tolerability profile. Focused psychotherapy and pharmacotherapy can have additive or complementary effects and, as such, may be better used in combination, particularly by patients with more advanced forms of TRD.

At present, there is no rational, evidence-based way to pick among the various cognitive, behavioural, interpersonal and time-limited psychodynamic therapies for a particular patient. Nevertheless, a systematic and transtheoretical approach that includes developing and maintaining a collaborative alliance, identifying, operationalizing and monitoring short-term goals, improving coping and self-management strategies to address persistent symptoms such as generalized anxiety, fatigue and insomnia and helping patients to tackle or at least lessen problems in everyday life is likely to improve the symptomatic and overall outcomes of people with TRD.

References

Basco, M. R. & Rush, A. J. (1995) Compliance of pharmacotherapy in mood disorders. *Psychiatric Ann.*, **25**, 269–270, 276–279.

Beck, A. T., Rush, A. J., Shaw, B. F. *et al.* (1979) *Cognitive Therapy of Depression: A Treatment Manual*, Guilford Press, New York, NY, USA.

Coffman, S. J., Martell, C. R., Dimidjian, S. *et al.* (2007) Extreme nonresponse in cognitive therapy: can behavioral activation succeed where cognitive therapy fails? *J. Cons. Clin. Psychol.*, **75**(4), 531–541.

Corey-Lisle, P. K., Nash, R., Stang, P. & Swindle, R. (2004) Response, partial response, and non-response in primary care treatment of depression. *Arch. Int. Med.*, **164**(11), 1197–1204.

Cuijpers, P., Dekker, J., Hollon, S. D. & Andersson, G. (2009) Adding psychotherapy to pharmacotherapy in the treatment of depressive disorders in adults: a meta-analysis. *J. Clin. Psychiatry*, **70**(9), 1219–1229.

Cuijpers, P., Geraedts, A. S., van Oppen, P. *et al.* (2011) Interpersonal psychotherapy for depression: a meta-analysis. *Am. J. Psychiatry*, **168**(6), 581–592.

Cuijpers, P., Smit, F., Bohlmeijer, E. *et al.* (2010) Efficacy of cognitive-behavioural therapy and other psychological treatments for adult depression: meta-analytic study of publication bias. *Brit. J. Psychiatry*, **196**(3), 173–178.

Cuijpers, P., Driessen, E., Hollon, S. D. *et al.* (2012) The efficacy of non-directive supportive therapy for adult depression: a meta-analysis. *Clin. Psychol. Rev.*, **32**(4), 280–291.

de Maat, S. M., Dekker, J., Schoevers, R. A. & de Jonghe, F. (2007) Relative efficacy of psychotherapy and combined therapy in the treatment of depression: a meta-analysis. *Eur. Psychiatry*, **22**(1), 1–8.

DeRubeis, R. J., Gelfand, L. A., Tang, T. Z. & Simons, A. D. (1999) Medications versus cognitive behavior therapy for severely depressed outpatients: mega-analysis of four randomized comparisons. *Am. J. Psychiatry*, **156**(7), 1007–1013.

DeRubeis, R. J., Hollon, S. D., Amsterdam, J. D. *et al.* (2005) Cognitive therapy vs medications in the treatment of moderate to severe depression. *Arch. Gen. Psychiatry*, **62**(4), 409–416.

Dimidjian, S., Hollon, S. D., Dobson, K. S. *et al.* (2006) Randomized trial of behavioral activation, cognitive therapy, and antidepressant medication in the acute treatment of adults with major depression. *J. Cons. Clin. Psychol.*, **74**(4), 658–670.

Dimidjian, S., Barrera, M. Jr, Martell, C. *et al.* (2011) The origins and current status of behavioral activation treatments for depression. *Ann. Rev. Clin. Psychol.*, **7**, 1–38.

Dobson, K. S., Hollon, S. D., Dimidjian, S. *et al.* (2008) Randomized trial of behavioral activation, cognitive therapy, and antidepressant medication in the prevention of relapse and recurrence in major depression. *J. Cons. Clin. Psychol.*, **76**(3), 468–477.

Driessen, E., Cuijpers, P., de Maat, S. C. *et al.* (2010a) The efficacy of short-term psychodynamic psychotherapy for depression: a meta-analysis. *Clin. Psychol. Rev.*, **30**(1), 25–36.

Driessen, E., Cuijpers, P., Hollon, S. D. & Dekker, J. J. (2010b) Does pretreatment severity moderate the efficacy of psychological treatment of adult outpatient depression? A meta-analysis. *J. Cons. Clin. Psychol.*, **78**(5), 668–680.

Eisendrath, S., Chartier, M. & McLane, M. (2011) Adapting mindfulness-based cognitive therapy for treatment-resistant depression: a clinical case study. *Cogn. Behav. Pract.*, **18**(3), 362–370.

Fava, G. A. & Visani, D. (2008) Psychosocial determinants of recovery in depression. *Dialog. Clin. Neurosci.*, **10**(4), 461–472.

Fava, M., Evins, A. E., Dorer, D. J. & Schoenfeld, D. A. (2003) The problem of the placebo response in clinical trials for psychiatric disorders: culprits, possible remedies, and a novel study design approach. *Psychother. Psychosom.*, **72**(3), 115–127.

Fournier, J. C., DeRubeis, R. J., Hollon, S. D. *et al.* (2010) Antidepressant drug effects and depression severity: a patient-level meta-analysis. *JAMA*, **303**(1), 47–53.

Gaynes, B. N., Lux, L. J., Lloyd, S. W. *et al.* (2011) *Nonpharmacologic Interventions for Treatment-Resistant Depression in Adults*, Agency for Healthcare Research and Quality, Rockville, MD, USA.

Goldapple, K., Segal, Z., Garson, C. *et al.* (2004) Modulation of cortical-limbic pathways in major depression: treatment-specific effects of cognitive behavior therapy. *Arch. Gen. Psychiatry*, **61**(1), 34–41.

Harley, R., Sprich, S., Safren, S. *et al.* (2008) Adaptation of dialectical behavior therapy skills training group for treatment-resistant depression. *J. Nerv. Ment. Dis.*, **196**(2), 136–143.

Hollon, S. D., Jarrett, R. B., Nierenberg, A. A. *et al.* (2005) Psychotherapy and medication in the treatment of adult and geriatric depression: which monotherapy or combined treatment? *J. Clin. Psychiatry*, **66**(4), 455–468.

Jakobsen, J. C., Hansen, J. L., Simonsen, S. *et al.* (2012a) Effects of cognitive therapy versus interpersonal psychotherapy in patients with major depressive disorder: a systematic review of randomized clinical trials with meta-analyses and trial sequential analyses. *Psychol. Med.*, **42**(7), 1343–1357.

Jakobsen, J. C., Hansen, J. L., Simonsen, E. & Gluud, C. (2012b) The effect of adding psychodynamic therapy to antidepressants in patients with major depressive disorder. A systematic review of randomized clinical trials with meta-analyses and trial sequential analyses. *J. Affect. Disord.*, **137**(1–3), 4–14.

Keller, M. B., McCullough, J. P., Klein, D. N. *et al.* (2000) A comparison of nefazodone, the cognitive behavioral-analysis system of psychotherapy, and their combination for the treatment of chronic depression. *N. Engl. J. Med.*, **342**, 1462–1470.

Kennedy, S. H., Konarski, J. Z., Segal, Z. V. *et al.* (2007) Differences in brain glucose metabolism between responders to CBT and venlafaxine in a 16-week randomized controlled trial. *Am. J. Psychiatry*, **164**(5), 778–788.

Klerman, G. L., Weissman, M. M., Rounsaville, B. J. *et al.* (1984) *Interpersonal Psychotherapy of Depression*, Basic Books, New York, NY, USA.

Kocsis, J. H., Gelenberg, A. J., Rothbaum, B. O. *et al.*: REVAMP Investigators (2009a) Cognitive behavioral analysis system of psychotherapy and brief supportive psychotherapy for augmentation of antidepressant nonresponse in chronic depression: the REVAMP Trial. *Arch. Gen. Psychiatry*, **66**(11), 1178–1188.

Kocsis, J. H., Leon, A. C., Markowitz, J. C. *et al.* (2009b) Patient preference as a moderator of outcome for chronic forms of major depressive disorder treated with nefazodone, cognitive behavioral analysis system of psychotherapy, or their combination. *J. Clin. Psychiatry*, **70**(3), 354–361.

Krupnick, J. L., Sotsky, S. M., Simmens, S. *et al.* (1996) The role of therapeutic alliance in psychotherapy and pharmacotherapy outcome: findings in the National Institute of Mental Health Treatment of Depression Collaborative Research Program. *J. Cons. Clin. Psychol.*, **64**, 532–539.

Luyten, P. & Blatt, S. J. (2012) Psychodynamic treatment of depression. *Psychiatr. Clin. North Am.*, **35**(1), 111–129.

Mitchell, A. J. (2006) Depressed patients and treatment adherence. *Lancet*, **367**(9528), 2041–2043.

Olfson, M., Marcus, S. C., Druss, B. *et al.* (2002) National trends in the outpatient treatment of depression. *JAMA*, **287**(2), 203–209.

Pampallona, S., Bollini, P., Tibaldi, G. *et al.* (2004) Combined pharmacotherapy and psychological treatment for depression: a systematic review. *Arch. Gen. Psychiatry*, **61**(7), 714–719.

Parikh, S. V., Segal, Z. V., Grigoriadis, S. *et al.*: Canadian Network for Mood and Anxiety Treatments (CANMAT) (2009) Canadian Network for Mood and Anxiety Treatments (CANMAT) clinical guidelines for the management of major depressive disorder in adults. II. Psychotherapy alone or in combination with antidepressant medication. *J. Affect. Disord.*, **117**(Suppl. 1), S15–25.

Roose, S. P. & Psychoanalytic Outcome Committee (2012) The development of a psychoanalytic outcome study: choices, conflicts, and consensus. *J. Am. Psychoanal. Assoc.*, **60**(2), 311–335.

Rush, A. J., Fava, M., Wisniewski, S. R. *et al.*: STAR*D Investigators Group (2004) Sequenced treatment alternatives to relieve depression (STAR*D), rationale and design. *Control Clin. Trials*, **25**(1), 119–142.

Rush, A. J., Trivedi, M. H., Wisniewski, S. R. *et al.* (2006) Acute and longer-term outcomes in depressed outpatients requiring one or several treatment steps: a STAR*D report. *Am. J. Psychiatry*, **163**(11), 1905–1917.

Schatzberg, A. F., Rush, A. J., Arnow, B. A. *et al.* (2005) Chronic depression: medication (nefazodone) or psychotherapy (CBASP) is effective when the other is not. *Arch. Gen. Psychiatry*, **62**(5), 513–520.

Schramm, E., van Calker, D., Dykierek, P. *et al.* (2007) An intensive treatment program of interpersonal psychotherapy plus pharmacotherapy for depressed inpatients: acute and long-term results. *Am. J. Psychiatry*, **164**(5), 768–777.

Schramm, E., Schneider, D., Zobel, I. *et al.* (2008) Efficacy of Interpersonal Psychotherapy plus pharmacotherapy in chronically depressed inpatients. *J. Affect. Disord.*, **109**(1–2), 65–73.

Shea, M. T., Elkin, I., Imber, S. D. *et al.* (1992) Course of depressive symptoms over follow-up: findings from the National Institute of Mental Health Treatment of Depression Collaborative Research Program. *Arch. Gen. Psychiatry*, **49**, 782–787.

Sherbourne, C., Schoenbaum, M., Wells, K. B. & Croghan, T. W. (2004) Characteristics, treatment patterns, and outcomes of persistent depression despite treatment in primary care. *Gen. Hosp. Psychiatry*, **26**(2), 106–114.

Souery, D., Oswald, P., Massat, I. *et al.* (2007) Clinical factors associated with treatment resistance in major depressive disorder: results from a European multicenter study. *J. Clin. Psychiatry*, **68**(7), 1062–1070.

Stimpson, N., Agrawal, N. & Lewis, G. (2002) Randomised controlled trials investigating pharmacological and psychological interventions for treatment-refractory depression. Systematic review. *Brit. J. Psychiatry*, **181**, 284–294.

Taylor, D., Carlyle, J. A., McPherson, S. *et al.* (2012) Tavistock Adult Depression Study (TADS), a randomised controlled trial of psychoanalytic psychotherapy for treatment-resistant/treatment-refractory forms of depression. *BMC Psychiatry*, **12**(1), 60.

Thase, M. E. (2011) The small specific effects of antidepressants in clinical trials: what do they mean to psychiatrists? *Curr. Psychiatry Rep.*, **13**(6), 476–482.

Thase, M. E. & Howland, R. (1994) Refractory depression: relevance of psychosocial factors and therapies. *Psychiatry Ann.*, **24**, 232–240.

Thase, M. E. & Kupfer, D. J. (1987) Characteristics of treatment resistant depression, in *Treating Resistant Depression* (ed. J. Zohar & R. H. Bellmaker), PMA Publishing, New York, NY, USA, pp. 23–45.

Thase, M. E., Greenhouse, J. B., Frank, E. *et al.* (1997) Treatment of major depression with psychotherapy or psychotherapy-pharmacotherapy combinations. *Arch. Gen. Psychiatry*, **54**, 1009–1015.

Thase, M. E., Friedman, E. S. & Howland, R. H. (2001) Management of treatment-resistant depression: psychotherapeutic perspectives. *J. Clin. Psychiatry*, **62**(Suppl. 18), 18–24.

Thase, M. E., Friedman, E. S., Biggs, M. M. *et al.* (2007) Cognitive therapy versus medication in augmentation and switch strategies as second-step treatments: a STAR*D report. *Am. J. Psychiatry*, **164**(5), 739–752.

Thase, M. E., Larsen, K. G. & Kennedy, S. H. (2011) Assessing the 'true' effect of active antidepressant therapy v. placebo in major depressive disorder: use of a mixture model. *Brit. J. Psychiatry*, **199**(6), 501–507.

Thoma, N. C., McKay, D., Gerber, A. J. *et al.* (2012) A quality-based review of randomized controlled trials of cognitive-behavioral therapy for depression: an assessment and metaregression. *Am. J. Psychiatry*, **169**(1), 22–30.

Trivedi, R. B., Nieuwsma, J. A., Williams, J. W. Jr & Baker, D. (2009) *Evidence Synthesis for Determining the Efficacy of Psychotherapy for Treatment Resistant Depression*, Department of Veterans Affairs, Washington, DC, USA.

van Beljouw, I. M., Verhaak, P. F., Cuijpers, P. *et al.* (2010) The course of untreated anxiety and depression, and determinants of poor one-year outcome: a one-year cohort study. *BMC Psychiatry*, **10**, 86.

Wiles, N., Thomas, L., Abel, A. *et al.* (2012) Cognitive behavioural therapy as an adjunct to pharmacotherapy for primary care based patients with treatment resistant depression: results of the CoBalT randomised controlled trial. *Lancet*, **380**(S0140–6736), 61 552–61 559.

Wisniewski, S. R., Fava, M., Trivedi, M. H. *et al.* (2007) Acceptability of second-step treatments to depressed outpatients: a STAR*D report. *Am. J. Psychiatry*, **164**(5), 753–760.

Wisniewski, S. R., Rush, A. J., Nierenberg, A. A. *et al.* (2009) Can phase III trial results of antidepressant medications be generalized to clinical practice? A STAR*D report. *Am. J. Psychiatry*, **166**(5), 599–607.

Index

Note: Page numbers in *italics* refer to Figures; those in **bold** to Tables.

Treatment-resistant Depression, First Edition. Edited by Siegfried Kasper
and Stuart Montgomery.
© 2013 John Wiley & Sons, Ltd. Published 2013 by John Wiley & Sons, Ltd.